Multivariable Analysis
A Practical Guide for Clinicians and Public Health Researchers

Why do you need this book?

Multivariable analysis is confusing! Whether you are performing your first research project or attempting to interpret the output from a multivariable model, you have undoubtedly found this to be true. Basic biostatistics books are of little or no help to you, since their coverage often stops short of multivariable analysis. However, existing multivariable analysis books are too dense with mathematical formulae and derivations and are not designed to answer your most basic questions. Is there a book that steps aside from the math and simply explains how to understand, perform, and interpret multivariable analyses?

Yes. *Multivariable Analysis: A Practical Guide for Clinicians and Public Health Researchers*, as this new edition is titled, is precisely the reference that will lead your way. In fact, Dr. Mitchell Katz has asked and answered all of your questions for you!

Why should I do multivariable analysis?

How do I choose which type of multivariable to use?

How many subjects do I need to do multivariable analysis?

What if I have repeated observations of the same persons?

Answers and detailed explanations to these questions and more are found in this book. Also, it is loaded with useful tips, summary charts, figures, and references.

If you are a medical student, resident, or clinician, *Multivariable Analysis: A Practical Guide for Clinicians and Public Health Researchers* will prove an indispensable guide through the confusing terrain of statistical analysis.

This third edition has been fully revised to build on the enormous success of its predecessors. New features include new sections on Poisson and negative binomial regression, proportional odds analysis, and multinomial logistic regression, and an expanded section on interpretation of residuals.

Praise for first edition

"This is the first nonmathematical book on multivariable analysis addressed to clinicians. Its range, organization, brevity, and clarity make it useful as a reference, a text, and a guide for self-study. This book *is* 'a practical guide for clinicians.'"

Leonard E. Braitman, Ph.D., *Annals of Internal Medicine*

Mitchell H. Katz is Clinical Professor of Medicine, Epidemiology and Biostatistics at the University of California, San Francisco; and Director of the Los Angeles Department of Health Services, Los Angeles, USA.

Multivariable Analysis

A Practical Guide for Clinicians and Public Health Researchers

Third Edition

Mitchell H. Katz

Department of Medicine, Epidemiology and
Biostatistics, University of California, USA

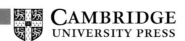

CAMBRIDGE
UNIVERSITY PRESS

CAMBRIDGE UNIVERSITY PRESS
Cambridge, New York, Melbourne, Madrid, Cape Town,
Singapore, São Paulo, Delhi, Tokyo, Mexico City

Cambridge University Press
The Edinburgh Building, Cambridge CB2 8RU, UK

Published in the United States of America by Cambridge University Press, New York

www.cambridge.org
Information on this title: www.cambridge.org/9780521760980

First published 1999
Second edition published 2006
Third edition published 2011

Printed in the United Kingdom at the University Press, Cambridge

A catalog record for this publication is available from the British Library

Library of Congress Cataloging in Publication data
Katz, Mitchell H., 1959– author.
    Multivariable analysis : a practical guide for clinicians and public health researchers /
    Mitchell H. Katz, Department of Medicine, Epidemiology, and Biostatistics,
    University of California, USA. – 3rd Edition.
        p. ; cm.
    Includes bibliographical references and index.
    ISBN 978-0-521-76098-0 (hardback) – ISBN 978-0-521-14107-9 (paperback)
    1. Medicine–Research–Statistical methods.   2. Multivariate analysis.   3. Biometry.
    4. Medical statistics.   I. Title.
    [DNLM: 1. Multivariate Analysis.   2. Biometry–methods. WA 950]
    R853.S7K38 2011
    610.72–dc22   2010052187

ISBN 978-0-521-76098-0 Hardback
ISBN 978-0-521-14107-9 Paperback

To my parents, for their unwavering support

Contents

Preface

There has been astounding growth in the use of multivariable analysis in clinical research. When the first edition of this book was published in 1999 logistic regression and proportional hazards models were cutting-edge techniques. Now for many researchers, these are old, staid models and the new edge is mixed-effects models, generalized estimating equations, Poisson regression, and propensity score analysis.

The use of these more sophisticated models is fueled by the development of user-friendly software for constructing multivariable models, increased availability of electronic databases (medical records, disease and procedure registries) that provide longitudinal data on large populations, and increased funding for and interest in clinical effectiveness studies – studies comparing different treatments in use – as a method of improving quality and reducing healthcare costs.

What hasn't changed in the past 11 years is the need for an easy-to-follow guide for nonstatisticians on how to perform and interpret these models. Although the available software (e.g., SPSS, SAS, S-plus, R) doesn't require programming experience or mathematical aptitude to conduct the analyses, if the analysis is not set up correctly, the answer is sure to be wrong! Even when the analysis is performed correctly, researchers may not draw the correct conclusions from the output.

To prevent these problems, throughout the book I have focused on how to set up and interpret multivariable analysis. I use examples from the medical and public health literature because illustrations of how to correctly analyze data and present the results will help you analyze and present your data correctly. Modeling your work based on successful published studies is one of the best and most efficient strategies for correctly analyzing data.

The biggest changes in this edition are that I have written new sections on Poisson and negative binomial regression, proportional odds analysis, and multinomial logistic regression because these models are increasingly in use. I have improved the section on mixed-effects models and generalized estimating equations, and also expanded the section on checking the underlying assumptions of multivariable models (Chapter 9) using residuals and other techniques.

While taking on new and more complicated material, I have maintained the basic organization of the book. Besides retaining the question-and-answer approach, the order of the book mirrors the process of doing multivariable analysis: deciding whether you need to do multivariable analysis (Chapters 1 and 2), choosing the correct model (Chapter 3), preparing your independent variables (Chapters 4 and 5), setting up the model (Chapter 6), performing the analysis (Chapter 7), interpreting the basic output (Chapter 8), delving deeper into the underlying assumptions of the model (Chapter 9), validating your model (Chapter 12) and publishing your study (Chapter 14). One of the reasons I prefer this approach to the more traditional approach (i.e., having a separate chapter on each type of multivariable model) is that it illustrates the similarities and differences of the different approaches. In my experience, when the results are strong, different (but reasonable) approaches lead to similar answers; conversely, when the results are very different with different techniques be suspicious. Also, I have found that the most efficient way to end an argument over what the best way is to analyze a data set is to analyze it multiple ways and see whether the results differ. If there are few differences then you have strengthened your results. When there are differences, you have probably learned something important about the nature of your data. Also, by structuring the book to parallel the research process, it allows readers to join the book at whatever stage they are at in the research process.

This book assumes that you are familiar with basic biostatistics. If not, I recommend S. Glantz's *Primer of Biostatistics* (sixth edition, McGraw-Hill, 2005). I have also written a basic statistics book using a question-and-answer approach similar to that used in this book called *Study Design and Statistical Analysis: A Practical Guide for Clinicians* (Cambridge University Press, 2006). Some reviewers have suggested that the two books be combined, and while I see the merit in that, I also see a much fatter text that might be more expensive and off-putting to clinical researchers. Please forgive me therefore if I cite that book or my other book on performing interventions (*Evaluating Clinical and Public Health Interventions*, Cambridge University Press, 2010). It is not an exercise of ego, but rather an attempt to keep each book inexpensive and short.

One of the challenges in writing a book for clinical researchers is deciding how much detail to include. One could easily have (and many have) written books larger than this about just one of the procedures described. To keep the presentations short and the material accessible, I direct readers who wish to know more about a particular procedure to more detailed sources in the footnotes. Since statistical textbooks are expensive, and many journal articles are not easy to find, I have particularly emphasized web resources that I have found useful.

Twenty years of students in the University of California, San Francisco, Clinical Research Program have contributed to this book through their insightful questions and observations. Serving as the Deputy Editor for the *Archives of Internal Medicine* during the past two years has definitely sharpened my eye as to how best to conduct multivariable research. For this opportunity I am grateful to the Editor, Rita Redberg, M.D., our two biostatistical editors who have taught me much, John Neuhaus, Ph.D. and David Glidden, Ph.D., and the other editors, Patrick O'Malley, M.D. and Kirsten Johansen, M.D., who have shared their critical observations with me on hundreds of articles. I greatly appreciate the support of my editor Richard Marley and the staff at Cambridge University Press for encouraging me to do this third edition.

The best part of writing and updating this book is the number of researchers who have emailed me with their comments, compliments, and questions. Writing textbooks is a lonely business and I wouldn't do it unless I had evidence that the books were actually helping people to conduct better research. If you have questions or suggestions for future editions, email me at mhkatz59@yahoo.com

Introduction

1.1 Why should I do multivariable analysis?

DEFINITION

Multivariable analysis is a tool for determining the relative contributions of different causes to a single event.

We live in a multivariable world. Most events, whether medical, political, social, or personal, have multiple causes. And these causes are related to one another. Multivariable analysis[1] is a statistical tool for determining the relative contributions of different causes to a single event or outcome.

Clinical researchers, in particular, need multivariable analysis because most diseases have multiple causes, and prognosis is usually determined by a large number of factors. Even for those infectious diseases that are known to be caused by a single pathogen, a number of factors affect whether an exposed individual becomes ill, including the characteristics of the pathogen (e.g., virulence of strain), the route of exposure (e.g., respiratory route), the intensity of exposure (e.g., size of inoculum), and the host response (e.g., immunologic defense).

Multivariable analysis allows us to sort out the multifaceted nature of risk factors and their relative contribution to outcome. For example, observational epidemiology has taught us that there are a number of risk factors associated with premature mortality, notably smoking, a sedentary lifestyle, obesity, elevated cholesterol, and hypertension. Note that I did not say that these factors *cause* premature mortality. Statistics alone cannot prove that a relationship between a risk factor and an outcome are causal.[2] Causality is established on

---

[1] The terms "multivariate analysis" and "multivariable analysis" are often used interchangeably. In the strict sense, multivariate analysis refers to simultaneously predicting multiple outcomes. Since this book deals with techniques that use multiple variables to predict a single outcome, I prefer the more general term multivariable analysis.

[2] Throughout the text I use the terms "associated with" and "related to" interchangeably. Similarly, I use the terms "risk factor," "exposure," "predictor," and "independent variable," and the terms "outcome" and "dependent variable," interchangeably. Although some of these terms such as "risk factor," "predictor," and "outcome" imply causality remember that causality can never be proven with statistical analysis. The best way for establishing causality is through rigorous study design (e.g., randomization to eliminate confounding, longitudinal observations to minimize the chance that the "outcome" caused the "risk factor").

the basis of biological plausibility and rigorous study designs, such as randomized controlled trials, which eliminate sources of potential bias.

Identification of risk factors of premature mortality through observational studies has been particularly important because you cannot randomize people to many of the conditions that cause premature mortality, such as smoking, sedentary lifestyle, or obesity. And yet these conditions tend to occur together; that is, people who smoke tend to exercise less and be more likely to be obese.

How does multivariable analysis separate the *independent* contribution of each of these factors? Let's consider the case of exercise. Numerous studies have shown that persons who exercise live longer than persons with sedentary lifestyles. But if the only reason that persons who exercise live longer is that they are less likely to smoke and more likely to eat low-fat meals leading to lower cholesterol, then initiating an exercise routine would not change a person's life expectancy.

The Aerobics Center Longitudinal Study tackled this important question.[3] They evaluated the relationship between exercise and mortality in 25,341 men and 7080 women. All participants had a baseline examination between 1970 and 1989. The examination included a physical examination, laboratory tests, and a treadmill evaluation to assess physical fitness. Participants were followed for an average of 8.4 years for the men and 7.5 years for the women.

Table 1.1 compares the characteristics of survivors to persons who had died during the follow-up. You can see that there are a number of significant differences between survivors and decedents among men and women. Specifically, survivors were younger, had lower blood pressure, lower cholesterol, were less likely to smoke, and were more physically fit (based on the length of time they stayed on the treadmill and their level of effort).

Although the results are interesting, Table 1.1 does not answer our basic question: Does being physically fit independently increase longevity? It doesn't answer the question because whereas the high-fitness group was less likely to die during the study period, those who were physically fit may just have been younger, been less likely to smoke, or had lower blood pressure.

To determine whether exercise is independently associated with mortality, the authors performed proportional hazards analysis, a type of multivariable analysis. The results are shown in Table 1.2. If you compare the number of deaths per thousand person-years in men, you can see that there were more

[3] Blair, S.N., Kampert, J.B., Kohl, H.W., *et al.* "Influences of cardiorespiratory fitness and other precursors on cardiovascular disease and all-cause mortality in men and women." *JAMA* **276** (1996): 205–10.

Table 1.1 Baseline characteristics of survivors and decedents, Aerobics Center Longitudinal Study.

| | Men | | Women | |
| | Survivors | Decedents | Survivors | Decedents |
Characteristics	(n = 24 740)	(n = 601)	(n = 6991)	(n = 89)
Age, y (SD)	42.7 (9.7)	52.1 (11.4)	42.6 (10.9)	53.3 (11.2)
Body mass index, kg/m^2 (SD)	26.0 (3.6)	26.3 (3.5)	22.6 (3.9)	23.7 (4.5)
Systolic blood pressure, mm Hg (SD)	121.1 (13.5)	130.4 (19.1)	112.6 (14.8)	122.6 (17.3)
Total cholesterol, mg/dL (SD)	213.1 (40.6)	228.9 (45.4)	202.7 (40.5)	228.2 (40.8)
Fasting glucose, mg/dL (SD)	100.4 (16.3)	108.1 (32.0)	94.4 (14.5)	99.9 (25.0)
Fitness, %				
Low	20.1	41.6	18.8	44.9
Moderate	42.0	39.1	40.6	33.7
High	37.9	19.3	40.6	21.3
Current or recent smoker, %	26.3	36.9	18.5	30.3
Family history of coronary heart disease, %	25.4	33.8	25.2	27.0
Abnormal electrocardiogram, %	6.9	26.3	4.8	18.0
Chronic illness, %	18.4	40.3	13.4	20.2

Adapted with permission from Blair, S. N., *et al.* "Influences of cardiorespiratory fitness and other precursors on cardiovascular disease and all-cause mortality in men and women." *JAMA* **276** (1996):205–10. Copyright 1996, American Medical Association. Additional data provided by authors.

deaths in the low-fitness group (38.1) than in the moderate/high fitness group (25.0). This difference is reflected in the elevated relative risk for lower fitness (38.1/25.0 = 1.52). These results are adjusted for all of the other variables listed in the table. This means that low fitness is associated with higher mortality, independent of the effects of other known risk factors for mortality, such as smoking, elevated blood pressure, cholesterol, and family history. A similar pattern is seen for women.

Was there any way to answer this question without multivariable analysis? One could have performed stratified analysis. Stratified analysis assesses the effect of a risk factor on outcome while holding another variable constant. So, for example, we could compare physically fit to unfit persons separately among smokers and nonsmokers. This would allow us to calculate a relative risk for the impact of fitness on mortality, independent of smoking. This analysis is shown in Table 1.3.

Unlike the multivariable analysis in Table 1.2, the analyses in Table 1.3 are bivariate.[4] We see that the mortality rate is greater among those at low fitness

DEFINITION

Stratified analysis assesses the effect of a risk factor on outcome while holding another variable constant.

---

[4] Some researchers use the term "univariate" to describe the association between two variables. I think it is more informative to restrict the term univariate to analyses of a single variable (e.g., mean, median), while using the term "bivariate" to refer to the association between two variables.

Table 1.2 Multivariable analysis of risk factors for all-cause mortality, Aerobics Center Longitudinal Study.

	Men		Women	
Independent variable	Deaths per 10 000 person-years	Adjusted relative risk (95% CI)	Deaths per 10 000 person-years	Adjusted relative risk (95% CI)
Fitness				
Low	38.1	1.52 (1.28–1.82)	27.8	2.10 (1.36–3.26)
Moderate/High	25.0	1.0 (ref.)	13.2	1.0 (ref.)
Smoking status				
Current or recent smoker	39.4	1.65 (1.39–1.97)	27.8	1.99 (1.25–3.17)
Past or never smoked	23.9	1.0 (ref.)	14.0	1.0 (ref.)
Systolic blood pressure				
$\geq$140 mm Hg	35.6	1.30 (1.08–1.58)	13.0	0.76 (0.41–1.40)
<140 mm Hg	27.3	1.0 (ref.)	17.1	1.0 (ref.)
Cholesterol				
$\geq$240 mg/dL	35.1	1.34 (1.13–1.59)	18.0	1.09 (0.68–1.74)
<240 mg/dL	26.1	1.0 (ref.)	16.6	1.0 (ref.)
Family history of coronary heart disease				
Yes	29.9	1.07 (0.90–1.29)	12.8	0.70 (0.43–1.16)
No	27.8	1.0 (ref.)	18.2	1.0 (ref.)
Body mass index				
$\geq$27 kg/m^2	28.8	1.02 (0.86–1.22)	15.9	0.94 (0.52–1.69)
<27 kg/m^2	28.2	1.0 (ref.)	16.9	1.0 (ref.)
Fasting glucose				
$\geq$120 mg/dL	34.4	1.24 (0.98–1.56)	29.6	1.79 (0.80–4.00)
<120 mg/dL	27.9	1.0 (ref.)	16.5	1.0 (ref.)
Abnormal electrocardiogram				
Yes	44.4	1.64 (1.34–2.01)	25.3	1.55 (0.87–2.77)
No	27.1	1.0 (ref.)	16.3	1.0 (ref.)
Chronic illness				
Yes	41.2	1.63 (1.37–1.95)	17.5	1.05 (0.61–1.82)
No	25.3	1.0 (ref.)	16.7	1.0 (ref.)

Adapted with permission from Blair, S. N., *et al.* "Influences of cardiorespiratory fitness and other precursors on cardiovascular disease and all-cause mortality in men and women." *JAMA* **276** (1996): 205–10. Copyright 1996, American Medical Association. Additional data provided by authors.

compared to those at moderate/high fitness, both among smokers (48.0 vs. 29.4) and among nonsmokers (44.0 vs. 20.1). This stratified analysis shows that the effect of fitness is independent of smoking status.

Table 1.3 Stratified analysis of smoking and fitness on all-cause mortality among men, Aerobics Center Longitudinal Study.

	Deaths per 10 000 person-years	Stratum-specific relative risk (95% CI)
Smokers		
Low fitness	48.0	1.63 (1.26–2.13)
Moderate/high fitness	29.4	1.0 (ref.)
Nonsmokers		
Low fitness	44.0	2.19 (1.77–2.70)
Moderate/high fitness	20.1	1.0 (ref.)

Data supplied by Aerobics Center Longitudinal Study.

But what about all of the other variables that might affect the relationship between fitness and longevity? You could certainly stratify for each one individually, proving that the effect of fitness on longevity is independent not only of smoking status, but also independent of elevated cholesterol, elevated blood pressure, and so on. However, this would only prove that the relationship is independent of these variables taken singly.

To stratify by two variables (smoking and cholesterol), you would have to assess the relationship between fitness and mortality in four groups (smokers with high cholesterol; smokers with low cholesterol; nonsmokers with high cholesterol; nonsmokers with low cholesterol). To stratify by three variables (smoking status, cholesterol level, and elevated blood pressure [yes/no]), you would have to assess the relationship between fitness and mortality in eight groups ($2 \times 2 \times 2 = 8$); add elevated glucose (yes/no) and you would have 16 groups ($2 \times 2 \times 2 \times 2 = 16$); add age (in six decades) and you would have 96 groups ($2 \times 2 \times 2 \times 2 \times 6 = 96$); and we haven't even yet taken into account all of the variables in Table 1.1 that are associated with mortality.

With each stratification variable you add, you increase the number of subgroups for which you have to individually assess whether the relationship between fitness and mortality holds. Besides producing mountains of printouts, and requiring a book (rather than a journal article) to report your results, you would likely have an insufficient sample size in some of these subgroups, even if you started with a large sample size. For example, in the Aerobics Center Longitudinal Study there were 25,341 men but only 601 deaths. With 96 subgroups, assuming uniform distributions, you would expect only about six deaths per subgroup. But, in reality, you wouldn't have uniform distributions. Some samples would be very small, and some would have no outcomes at all.

Multivariable analysis overcomes this limitation. It allows you to simultaneously assess the impact of multiple independent variables on outcome. But there is (always) a cost: The model makes certain assumptions about the nature of the data. These assumptions are sometimes hard to verify. We will take up these issues in Chapters 3, 4, and 9.

1.2 What are confounders and how does multivariable analysis help me to deal with them?

The ability of multivariable analysis to *simultaneously* assess the independent contribution of a number of risk factors to outcome is particularly important when you have "confounding." Confounding occurs when the apparent association between a risk factor and an outcome is affected by the relationship of a third variable to the risk factor and the outcome; the third variable is called a confounder.

> **DEFINITION**
>
> A *confounder* is associated with the risk factor and causally related to the outcome.

For a variable to be a confounder, the variable must be associated with the risk factor and causally related to the outcome (Figure 1.1).

A classically taught example of confounding is the relationship between carrying matches and developing lung cancer (Figure 1.2). Persons who carry matches have a greater chance of developing lung cancer; the confounder is smoking. This example is often used to illustrate confounding because it is easy to grasp that carrying matches cannot possibly cause lung cancer.

Stratified analysis can be used to assess and eliminate confounding. If you stratify by smoking status you will find that carrying matches is not associated with lung cancer. That is, there will be no relationship between carrying matches and lung cancer when you look separately among smokers and non-smokers (Figure 1.2). The statistical evidence of confounding is the difference

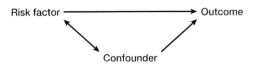

Figure 1.1   Relationships among risk factor, confounder, and outcome.

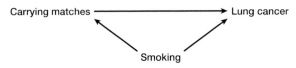

Figure 1.2   Relationships among carrying matches, smoking, and lung cancer.

between the unstratified and the stratified analysis. In the unstratified analysis the chi-squared test would be significant and the odds ratio for the impact of matches on lung cancer would be significantly greater than one. In the two stratified analyses (smokers and nonsmokers), carrying matches would not be significantly associated with lung cancer; the odds ratio would be one in both strata. This differs from the example of stratified analysis in Table 1.3 where exercise was significantly associated with mortality for both smokers and nonsmokers.

Most clinical examples of confounding are more subtle and harder to diagnose than the case of matches and lung cancer. Let's look at the relationship between smoking and prognosis in patients with coronary artery disease following angioplasty (the opening of clogged coronary vessels with the use of a wire and a balloon).

Everyone knows (although the cigarette companies long claimed ignorance) that smoking increases the risk of death. Countless studies, including the Aerobics Center Longitudinal Study (Table 1.2), have demonstrated that smoking is associated with increased mortality. How then can we explain the results of Hasdai and colleagues?[5] They followed 5437 patients with coronary artery disease, who had angioplasty. They divided their sample into nonsmokers, former smokers (quit at least six months before procedure), recent quitters (quit immediately following the procedure), and persistent smokers. The relative risk of death with the 95 percent confidence intervals are shown in Table 1.4.

How can the risk of death be lower among persons who persistently smoke than those who never smoked? In the case of recent quitters, you would expect their risk of death to return toward normal only after years of not smoking – and even then you wouldn't actually expect quitters to have a lower risk of death than nonsmokers.

Before you assume that there is something wrong with this study, several other studies have found a similar relationship between smoking and better prognosis among patients with coronary artery disease after thrombolytic therapy. This effect has been named the "smoker's paradox."[6] What is behind the paradox? Look at Table 1.5. As you can see, compared to nonsmokers and

[5] Hasdai, D., Garratt, K. N., Grill, D. E., *et al.* "Effect of smoking status on the long-term outcome after successful percutaneous coronary revascularization." *N. Engl. J. Med.* **336** (1997): 755–61.

[6] Barbash, G. I., Reiner, J., White, H. D., *et al.* "Evaluation of paradoxical beneficial effects of smoking in patients receiving thrombolytic therapy for acute myocardial infarction: Mechanisms of the 'smoker's paradox' from the GUSTO-I trial, with angiographic insights." *J. Am. Coll. Cardiol.* **26** (1995): 1222–9.

Table 1.4 Bivariate association between smoking status and risk of death.

Bivariate	Nonsmokers	Former smokers	Recent quitters	Persistent smokers
Relative risk of death	1.0 (ref.)	1.08 (0.92–1.26)	0.56 (0.40–0.77)	0.74 (0.59–0.94)

Adapted from Hasdai, D., *et al.* "Effect of smoking status on the long-term outcome after successful percutaneous coronary revascularization." *N. Engl. J. Med.* **336** (1997): 755–61.

Table 1.5 Association between demographic and clinical factors and smoking status.

	Nonsmokers	Former smokers	Recent quitters	Persistent smokers
Age, year ± SD	67 ± 11	65 ± 10	56 ± 10	55 ± 11
Duration of angina, months ± SD	41 ± 66	51 ± 72	21 ± 46	29 ± 55
Diabetes, %	21%	18%	8%	10%
Hypertension, %	54%	48%	38%	39%
Extent of coronary artery disease, %				
One vessel	50%	51%	57%	55%
Two vessels	36%	36%	34%	36%
Three vessels	14%	13%	10%	9%

Adapted from Hasdai, D., *et al.* "Effect of smoking status on the long-term outcome after successful percutaneous coronary revascularization." *N. Engl. J. Med.* **336** (1997): 755–61.

former smokers, quitters and persistent smokers are younger, have had angina for a shorter period of time, are less likely to have diabetes and hypertension, and have less severe coronary artery disease (i.e., more one-vessel disease and less three-vessel disease). Given this, it is not so surprising that the recent quitters and persistent smokers have a lower risk of death than nonsmokers and former smokers: They are younger and have fewer underlying medical problems than the nonsmokers and former smokers.

Compare the bivariate (unadjusted) risk of death to the multivariable risk of death (Table 1.6). Note that in the multivariable analysis the researchers adjusted for those differences, such as age and duration of angina, that existed among the four groups.

With statistical adjustment for the baseline differences between the groups, the former smokers and persistent smokers have a significantly greater risk of death than nonsmokers – a much more sensible result. (The recent quitters also have a greater risk of death than the nonsmokers, but the confidence intervals of the relative risk do not exclude one.) The difference between the bivariate and multivariable analysis indicates that confounding is present. The advantage of multivariable analysis over stratified analysis is that it would

> **TIP**
>
> Multivariable analysis is preferable to stratified analysis when you have multiple confounders.

Table 1.6 Comparison of bivariate and multivariable association between smoking status and risk of death.

	Nonsmokers	Former smokers	Recent quitters	Persistent smokers
Relative risk of death (bivariate)	1.0 (ref.)	1.08 (0.92–1.26)	0.56 (0.40–0.77)	0.74 (0.59–0.94)
Relative risk of death (multivariable)	1.0 (ref.)	1.34 (1.14–1.57)	1.21 (0.87–1.70)	1.76 (1.37–2.26)

Adapted from Hasdai, D., *et al*. "Effect of smoking status on the long-term outcome after successful percutaneous coronary revascularization." *N. Engl. J. Med.* **336** (1997): 755–61.

have been difficult to stratify for age, duration of angina, diabetes, hypertension, and extent of coronary artery disease.

1.3 What are suppressers and how does multivariable analysis help me to deal with them?

> **TIP**
>
> Unlike a typical confounder, when you have a suppresser you won't see any bivariate association between the risk factor and the outcome until you adjust for the suppresser.

Suppresser variables are a type of confounder. As with confounders, a suppresser is associated with the risk factor and the outcome (Figure 1.3). The difference is that on bivariate analysis there is no effect seen between the risk factor and the outcome. But when you adjust for the suppresser, the relationship between the risk factor and the outcome becomes significant.

Identifying and adjusting for suppressers can lead to important findings. For example, it was unknown whether taking antiretroviral treatment would prevent HIV seroconversion among healthcare workers who sustained a needle stick from a patient who was HIV-infected. For several years, healthcare workers who had an exposure were offered zidovudine treatment, but they were told that there was no efficacy data to support its use. A randomized controlled trial was attempted, but it was disbanded because healthcare workers did not wish to be randomized.

Since a randomized controlled trial was not possible, a case-control study was performed instead.[7] The cases were healthcare workers who sustained a needle stick and had seroconverted. The controls were healthcare workers who sustained a needle stick but had remained HIV-negative. The question was whether the proportion of persons taking zidovudine would be lower in the group who had seroconverted (the cases) than in the group who had not become infected (the controls). The investigators found that the proportion of cases using zidovudine was lower (9 of 33 cases or 27 percent) than the

[7] Cardo, D. M., Culver, D. H., Ciesielski, C. A., *et al.* "A case-control study of HIV seroconversion in health-care workers after percutaneous exposure." *N. Engl. J. Med.* **337** (1997): 1485–90.

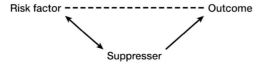

Figure 1.3   Relationships among risk factor, suppresser, and outcome.

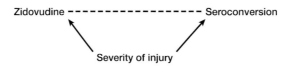

Figure 1.4   Relationships among zidovudine, severity of injury, and seroconversion.

proportion of controls using zidovudine (247 of 679 controls or 36 percent), but the difference was not statistically significant (probability [P] = 0.35). Consistent with this nonsignificant trend, the odds ratio shows that zidovudine was protective (0.7), but the 95 percent confidence intervals were wide and did not exclude one (0.3–1.4).

However, it was known that healthcare workers who sustained an especially serious exposure (e.g., a deep injury or who stuck themselves with a needle that had visible blood on it) were more likely to choose to take zidovudine than healthcare workers who had more minor exposures. Also, healthcare workers who had serious exposures were more likely to seroconvert.

When the researchers adjusted their analysis for severity of injury using multiple logistic regression, zidovudine use was associated with a significantly lower risk of seroconversion (odds ratio [OR] = 0.2; 95 percent confidence interval (CI) = 0.1 – 0.6; $P < 0.01$). Thus, we have an example of a suppresser effect as shown in Figure 1.4. Severity of exposure is associated with zidovudine use and causally related to seroconversion. Zidovudine use is not associated with seroconversion in bivariate analyses but becomes significant when you adjust for severity of injury.

Although this multivariable analysis demonstrated the efficacy of zidovudine on preventing seroconversion by incorporating the suppresser variables, it should be remembered that multivariable analysis cannot adjust for other potential biases in the analysis. For example, the cases and controls for this study were not chosen from the same population, raising the possibility that selection bias may have influenced the results. Nonetheless, on the strength of this study, postexposure prophylaxis with antiretroviral treatment became the standard of care for healthcare workers who sustained needle sticks from HIV-contaminated needles.

1.4 What are interactions and how does multivariable analysis help me to deal with them?

DEFINITION

An *interaction* occurs when the impact of a risk factor on outcome is changed by the value of a third variable.

An interaction occurs when the impact of a risk factor on outcome is changed by the value of a third variable. Interaction is sometimes referred to as effect modification, since the effect of the risk factor on outcome is modified by another variable.

An interaction is illustrated in Figure 1.5. The risk factor's effect on outcome (solid lines) differs depending on the value of the interaction variable (whether it is 1 or 0). The dotted line indicates the relationship without consideration of the interaction effect.

In extreme cases, an interaction may completely reverse the relationship between the risk factor and the outcome. This would occur when the risk factor increased the likelihood of outcome at one value of the interaction variable but decreased the likelihood of outcome at a different value of the interaction variable. More commonly, the effect of the risk factor on the outcome is stronger (or weaker) at certain values of the third variable.

As with confounding, stratification can be used to identify an interaction. By stratifying by the interaction variable, you can observe the effect of a risk factor on outcome at the different values of the interaction variable. You can statistically test whether the association between a risk factor and an outcome at different levels of the interaction variable are statistically different from one another using a chi-squared test for homogeneity.

However, as with the use of stratification to eliminate confounding, use of stratification to demonstrate interaction has limitations. It is cumbersome to stratify by more than one or two variables; yet you may have multiple interactions in your data. Whereas stratification will accurately quantify the effect of the risk factor on the outcome at different levels of the interaction variable, this analysis will not be adjusted for the other variables in your model (e.g., confounders) that may affect the relationship between risk factor and outcome. Multivariable analysis allows you

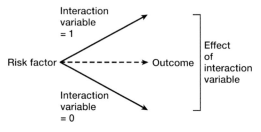

Figure 1.5   Illustration of an interaction effect.

Table 1.7 Association of independent variables with confirmed diagnosis of acute myocardial infarction based on multiple logistic regression model.

Independent variables	Coefficients	Odds ratio
Male gender	**0.4852**	**1.6**
Age <50	0.1432	1.2
Chest pain	0.8792	2.4
Chief complaint: chest pain	0.4399	1.6
Nausea/vomiting	0.5153	1.7
Congestive heart failure	0.6759	2.0
White race	0.0987	1.1
ST elevation	**2.0948**	**8.1**
ST depression	1.2632	3.5
Q waves	0.5311	1.7
History of diabetes mellitus	0.2781	1.3
History of hypertension	0.2032	1.2
History of angina	−0.2976	0.7
History of peptic ulcers	−0.3210	0.7
Dizziness	−0.4437	0.6
Interactions		
Male gender and congestive heart failure	−0.6899	0.5
Male gender and ST elevation	**−0.5187**	**0.6**
Male gender and white race	0.5206	1.7

Adapted with permission from Zucker, D.R., *et al.* "Presentations of acute myocardial infarction in men and women." *J. Gen. Intern. Med.* **12** (1997): 79–87.

to include interaction terms and assess them while adjusting for other variables.

For example, Zucker and colleagues evaluated whether specific signs or symptoms of myocardial infarction were different in men than in women presenting to the emergency department with chest pain or other symptoms of acute cardiac ischemia.[8]

In Table 1.7 you can see the association between the independent variables and confirmed diagnoses of acute myocardial infarction. The coefficients and odds ratios are from a multiple logistic regression model. The authors found three significant interactions involving gender: male gender and ST elevation (on electrocardiogram), male gender and congestive heart failure, and male gender and white race.

[8] Zucker, D.R., Griffith, J.L., Beshansky, J.R., *et al.* "Presentations of acute myocardial infarction in men and women." *J. Gen. Intern. Med.* **12** (1997): 79–87.

What do these interactions mean? Let's use the interaction involving male gender and ST elevations as an example (I have put these two variables and their interaction term in bold print). Note that men were more likely than women to have an acute myocardial infarction (OR = 1.6), even after adjusting for other variables associated with an infarction. Similarly, ST elevations were more likely to indicate ischemia (OR = 8.1). Given this, you would expect that males with ST elevations would have a markedly higher risk of myocardial infarction ($1.6 \times 8.1 = 13.0$) than women ($1.0 \times 8.1 = 8.1$) (the wonderful property of odds ratios that allows you to multiply them this way is explained in Section 9.7).

The multiplication of the odds ratios of gender and ST elevations would lead you to believe that men with ST elevations would have a significantly higher risk of an acute myocardial infarction than women (13.0 vs. 8.1). In fact, the risk for men and women with ST elevations was similar. This is reflected in the negative coefficient for male gender $\times$ ST elevations and the odds ratio of 0.6. If you multiply out the odds ratio for the interaction of male gender with ST elevations, men with ST elevations ($1.6 \times 8.1 \times 0.6 = 7.8$) and women with ST elevations ($1.0 \times 8.1 \times 1.0 = 8.1$) have a similar risk of myocardial infarction.

ST elevations are highly specific for (although not diagnostic of) myocardial infarction. It is not surprising, therefore, that the risks of myocardial infarction are similar in men and women with ST elevations. Had being male made it even worse to have ST elevations the coefficient would have been positive, the odds ratio would have been greater than one, and we would have seen an even greater difference between the risk of an acute myocardial infarction for men and for women in the presence of ST elevations than the difference between 13.0 and 8.1.

Because interaction effects can be difficult to assess and interpret, I will return to this topic in Sections 7.3, 8.4, and 9.7.

Common uses of multivariable models

2.1 What are the most common uses of multivariable models in clinical research?

The four most common uses of multivariable models are:

A observational studies of etiology
B intervention studies (randomized and nonrandomized)
C studies of diagnosis
D studies of prognosis

These different uses are discussed in the Sections 2.2–2.5.

2.2 How is multivariable analysis used in observational studies of etiology?

The goal of etiologic studies is to identify *causes* of an outcome, usually with the goal of removing a harmful substance (e.g., tobacco) or promoting a healthful activity (e.g., exercise).

Although observational studies cannot prove causality, multivariable analysis may strengthen the argument for causality by excluding confounding, an alternative explanation of an association. Look back at the example of fitness and mortality in Chapter 1. If the association between fitness and longevity is causal, encouraging people to exercise more will extend their life. If the association between fitness is confounded by smoking (i.e., smoking is the real cause of the decreased lifespan, and because smokers exercise less it appears that fitness is associated with longevity) increasing fitness will not change longevity. The data in Table 1.2 indicate that the effect of fitness on longevity is not confounded by smoking or other factors (at least not the ones the authors adjusted for) and therefore fitness programs are a promising intervention for extending survival.

Part of why multivariable analysis has become indispensable to observational studies of etiology is that as we have learned more about certain multifactorial diseases, such as cardiac disease, we have identified a larger and larger number of risk factors for the disease. Because many of these variables are associated with one another, stratification becomes an unwieldy technique for eliminating confounding. For example, when Gardner and colleagues assessed whether the size of low-density lipoprotein particles affected the incidence of coronary artery disease they adjusted their analysis for those risk factors long known to increase the risk of coronary artery disease, such as smoking, blood pressure, and body mass index.[1] But they also adjusted their model for more recently identified risk factors such as HDL cholesterol, nonHDL cholesterol, and triglycerides. One of the most extensive studies of cardiovascular disease, the Framingham study, which began in 1948, did not even collect data on HDL cholesterol until 1972.[2]

> It is impossible to adjust for those variables that are unmeasured or unknown!

Unfortunately multivariable analysis has limitations when used for observational studies of etiology. Perhaps the greatest one is that it is impossible to adjust for those variables that are unmeasured or unknown! Therefore, even after you have adjusted for all those variables that have been measured, there remains the possibility that the association is still confounded.

A second limitation of multivariable analysis is that including a potential confounder in a model does not guarantee elimination of bias owing to the confounder. For multivariable models to adequately adjust for confounding, there must be sufficient overlap of the confounders in the different groups or outcomes. For example, if almost all of the smokers are in one group and almost all of the nonsmokers are in another group, adjusting for smoking will not remove confounding caused by smoking. This is why it is important to use bivariate analysis to verify that there is sufficient overlap of your potential confounders prior to conducting a multivariable analysis.

> **TIP**
>
> Prior to conducting multivariable analysis, use bivariate analysis to verify that there is sufficient overlap of your potential confounders.

Even if there is sufficient overlap, no adjustment is perfect. Just as there is error in the measurement of your dependent and independent variables, there is error in your confounders. Once you appreciate that your measurement of confounding variables is imperfect, you realize that including a variable in a model cannot completely eliminate confounding. Moreover, the models themselves contain error. Important variables may be omitted, they may be incorrectly specified (Section 4.3), or interactions between the variables may not

---

[1] Gardner, C. D., Fortmann, S. P., and Krauss, R. M. "Association of small low-density lipoprotein particles with the incidence of coronary artery disease in men and women." *JAMA* **276** (1996): 875–81.

[2] Levy, D., Wilson, P. W. F., Anderson, K. M., *et al.* "Stratifying the patient at risk from coronary disease: New insights from the Framingham heart study." *Am. Heart. J.* **119** (1990): 712–17.

be appropriately accounted for (Section 9.7). This warning is not meant to be discouraging; rather, it is stated to promote humility about what you can and cannot do with statistical models.

2.3 How is multivariable analysis used in intervention studies (randomized and nonrandomized)?

When analyzing data from intervention trials, whether the trials are randomized or nonrandomized, whether the intervention is a drug, a counseling session, or a change in law, it is critical to adjust for baseline differences in the groups. Why? Because if the groups being compared are different at the start of the study it is impossible to know whether differences between the groups at the end of the study are owing to the intervention or are owing to the inherent differences between the groups. For example, what if those who received a drug were older than those who received a placebo, or if those who received a counseling session were more educated than those who received usual care, or if those living in a state that passed a law have higher incomes than those living in a state that did not pass the same? In all these cases it will be impossible to know whether any differences between the groups at the end of the study are owing to the intervention or these baseline differences.

> **TIP**
>
> When there are baseline differences between groups in an intervention study it is impossible to know whether differences between the groups at the end of the study are owing to the intervention or owing to the inherent differences between the groups.

In nonrandomized intervention studies, substantial differences between the groups at baseline are the rule, rather than the exception. In the real world people do not randomly allocate themselves. People on medicines are likely to be sicker, or have better access to medical care, or have more aggressive physicians than people who are not taking medicines. People who sign up for counseling sessions are likely to be more motivated about their health than those receiving usual care. People living in states that pass certain laws are likely different from people living in other states.

None of this should discourage you from conducting nonrandomized intervention trials. In fact there are many instances when expense, logistical, or ethical difficulties preclude randomizing patients. In such cases multivariable analysis can be used to statistically approximate comparable groups.

> **TIP**
>
> When randomization is impossible, use multivariable analysis to statistically approximate equal comparison groups.

Multivariable analysis was used to adjust for known confounders in an important nonrandomized study of statin therapy in patients admitted to hospital with acute coronary syndromes (i.e., symptoms and signs of ischemia).[3] The investigators compared 5959 patients who were begun on statin treatment during hospitalization to 9522 patients who were not. They found that

---

[3] Spencer, F. A., Allegrone, J., Goldberg, R. J., *et al.* "Association of statin therapy with outcomes of acute coronary syndromes: The Grace study." *Ann. Intern. Med.* **140** (2004): 857–66.

patients treated with statins were significantly less likely to die in the hospital (OR = 0.19; 95% CI = 0.16 – 0.23).

Does this bivariate analysis prove that statins decrease death owing to acute coronary syndromes? No! Since treatment was not randomized, it is likely that there were important differences between patients who received statin treatment in the hospital and those who did not. Indeed, as you can see from Table 2.1, patients receiving statin therapy were different from those who did not receive it, in terms of their demographics, medical history, presenting characteristics, long-term medications, in-hospital medications, and interventions. Perhaps it is these differences that resulted in patients who were treated with statins being less likely to die.

To adjust for these baseline differences, the authors performed a multivariable analysis. With adjustment for differences in demographics, medical history, presenting characteristics, long-term medications, in-hospital medications, and interventions, statin use was still significantly associated with a decreased likelihood of death (OR = 0.38; 95 % CI = 0.30 – 0.48). The fact that the adjusted odds ratio is somewhat higher than the bivariate odds ratio indicates that there was confounding. But even after adjustment for multiple confounders, statin use does have an independent effect on reducing mortality in patients with acute coronary syndromes.

The major limitation of this study is the same as the major limitation of all nonrandomized intervention studies. Multivariable analysis cannot adjust for unknown or unmeasured confounders – so if there is some other difference between those patients who were receiving statins and those patients who were not and this difference was associated with mortality then the use of statins may not be the true cause of the decreased mortality. Only randomization can create groups that are equal with respect to both measured and unmeasured confounders.

Figure 2.1 illustrates the elegance of randomization. If group assignment is determined through a *nonbiased* randomization, there is no association between a potential confounder and group assignment. I put nonbiased in italics to remind you that the advantages of randomization are lost if bias creeps in. This can occur if, for example, a research assistant knows which group the next person enrolled in the study will be assigned to and therefore seeks to enroll a particular patient next. This is why randomization should be done by someone with no contact or extraneous information about the subject.

Unfortunately, even when randomization occurs without bias, it sometimes happens by chance that one group is different from another group. For example, Mittelman and colleagues conducted an intervention to delay

---

TIP

The advantage of randomization is that you can never adjust for what you don't know or can't measure.

Randomization produces nonbiased comparisons groups.

Sometimes by chance there are important differences between randomized groups.

Table 2.1 Differences between patients who received statin treatment in the hospital and those who did not.

Characteristic	In-hospital statin use ($n = 5959$)	No statin use ($n = 9522$)	P Value
Demographic			
Median age, y	62.7	69.8	<0.001
Women, %	29.6	36.7	<0.001
Medical history, %			
Smoking	63.7	52.6	<0.001
Myocardial infarction	19.6	28.2	<0.001
Transient ischemic attack or stroke	5.6	9.4	<0.001
Diabetes	20.1	23.7	<0.001
Positive angiogram	15.5	20.2	<0.001
Peripheral vascular disease	7.5	9.9	<0.001
Hypertension	52.1	58.7	<0.001
Hyperlipidemia	43.0	25.0	<0.001
Percutaneous coronary intervention	8.0	9.6	<0.001
Coronary artery bypass graft surgery	6.4	9.5	<0.001
Presenting characteristics, %			
Killip class			
I	86.2	76.7	<0.001
II	10.8	16.3	
III	2.5	5.3	
IV	0.5	1.7	
Heart rate ≥100 beats/min	13.8	19.5	<0.001
Systolic blood pressure <90 mm Hg	1.6	3.2	<0.001
ST-segment elevation	49	36.7	<0.001
Other long-term medication, %			
Aspirin	26.9	36.2	<0.001
ACE inhibitors	17	24.9	<0.001
β-blockers	17.5	24.1	<0.001
Other lipid-lowering agents	2.4	2.6	>0.2
Other in-hospital medication, %			
Aspirin	96.6	90.9	<0.001
Ticlopidine or clopidogrel	46.9	25.9	<0.001
Unfractionated heparin	53.5	49.9	<0.001
Enoxaparin	48.3	38.5	<0.001
Other low-molecular-weight heparin	12.9	9.6	<0.001

Characteristic	In-hospital statin use ($n = 5959$)	No statin use ($n = 9522$)	P Value
ACE inhibitor	64.8	56.7	<0.001
β-blockers	85.9	71.4	<0.001
Other lipid-lowering agents	2.1	4.6	<0.001
Glycoprotein IIb/IIIa inhibitors	27.1	13.2	<0.001
Interventions, %			
Cardiac catheterization	59.9	41.7	<0.001
Percutaneous coronary intervention	40.9	22.8	<0.001
Coronary artery bypass graft surgery	5.4	5.3	>0.2

Data from: Spencer, F. A., Allegrone, J., Goldberg, R. J., *et al.* "Association of statin therapy with outcomes of acute coronary syndromes: The Grace study." *Ann. Intern. Med.* **140** (2004): 857–66.

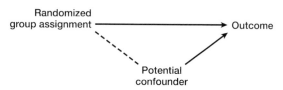

Figure 2.1   Relationships among randomized group assignment, potential confounder, and outcome.

nursing-home placement of patients with Alzheimer's disease.[4] They randomized families to a treatment group (counseling and support for caregivers) and a control group. By chance (and bad luck!), the primary caregiver was significantly more likely to be female among the families randomized to the control group than among the families randomized to the treatment group. Moreover, patients of female caregivers were significantly more likely to be placed in a nursing home (the main outcome of this study). Thus, without adjustment for the gender of the caregiver, the results of the study would have been difficult to interpret. With adjustment for the gender of the caregiver, the authors demonstrated that the treatment was associated with a decrease in nursing-home placement.

[4] Mittelman, M. S., Ferris, S. H., Shulman, E., *et al.* "A family intervention to delay nursing home placement of patients with Alzheimer disease." *JAMA* **276** (1996): 1725–31.

In the case of this study, the difference in the baseline variable (gender of primary caregiver) was statistically significant. However, even if none of the differences is statistically significant, smaller differences between the groups may raise questions as to whether the baseline groups really are comparable. Therefore, with randomized trials most investigators will test the effect of their intervention using both bivariate and multivariable analyses. When bivariate and multivariable results are similar, this is strong evidence that there is not confounding, at least not owing to those variables included in the model. When bivariate and multivariable results are different in a randomized study the results are harder to interpret, in part because statistical adjustment introduces model error. Thus if your randomized clinical trial shows no or only a borderline effect in the bivariate analysis but a statistically significant effect in the multivariable analysis, some readers will be suspicious that the apparent effect is actually owing to error in the model.

Another use of multivariable analysis in randomized controlled trials is to determine whether other factors besides treatment group are associated with outcome. This use is akin to using multivariable analysis to determine etiologic risk factors in an observational study (Section 2.2); even though the study is "randomized", subjects are not randomized on the factors other than the main intervention.

For example, Swain and colleagues conducted a randomized trial to determine whether concurrent or sequential chemotherapy would be better for women with operable, lymph-node-positive breast cancer.[5] The women were randomized to three different groups. Those randomized to sequential chemotherapy did the best, answering the main question of the study. However, a secondary aim of the study was to determine the association between amenorrhea (loss of menstrual periods for at least six months) and survival. Using a proportional hazards analysis the investigators found that survival was significantly longer among women who had amenorrhea than those who did not (relative hazard 0.76; P value = 0.4). The analysis was adjusted for treatment assignment, estrogen-receptor status, age, lymph-node status, tumor size, and use of hormone therapy. It is important to understand that this is an independent effect of amenorrhea and not an interaction (Section 1.4). The authors explicitly checked to see if there was an interaction between developing amenorrhea and treatment assignment, estrogen-receptor status,

---

[5] Swain, S. M., Jeong, J., Geyer, C. E., *et al.* "Longer therapy, iatrogenic amenorrhea, and survival in early breast cancer." *N. Engl. J. Med.* **362** (2010): 2053–65.

and age, and found that the effect of amenorrhea was consistent across all subgroups analyzed.

2.4 How is multivariable analysis used in studies of diagnosis?

Multivariable models can identify the best combination of diagnostic information to determine whether a person has a particular disease. The most extensive work on diagnostic algorithms has been done for determining the likelihood of a myocardial infarction in patients presenting to emergency departments with chest pain. The reason this question has received so much attention is that the stakes are high. Chest pain is a common presenting symptom in the emergency department. It can be due to something as minor as heartburn or something as serious as a heart attack. Every day, in every emergency department, clinicians decide whom to send home and whom to admit to the coronary care unit. Although coronary care units save lives for patients with acute ischemia, less than half of those receiving this costly intervention actually have ischemia. There is no one test available at the time of an emergency-department visit that distinguishes those patients who should be admitted from those who could be sent home.

> **TIP**
>
> Use multivariable models to determine the best combination of diagnostic information.

Pozen and colleagues developed a diagnostic model for determining the likelihood that a patient presenting to an emergency department with chest pain had acute ischemia.[6] From 59 different clinical features they identified seven clinical features that, when used together in a logistic regression model, produced a prediction of ischemia from 0 to 1.0. To determine the usefulness of the model, the researchers gave the results (during the experimental period) to treating physicians before they had to determine whether to admit patients or send them home. During the control period, the physicians were not given the estimates of the probability of acute ischemia. The researchers found that when the physicians were given the information, their decision-making improved. In particular, the number of coronary-care-unit admissions decreased by 30 percent without any missed cases of ischemia.

So when confronted with a patient with chest pain, do most emergency department physicians whip out their hand-held calculator and compute the probability of ischemia? Sadly, no. Corey and Merenstein tested the acceptability of this model to physicians by providing a worksheet version of the algorithm in a convenient dispenser in the emergency department, but not

---

[6] Pozen, M. W., D'Agostino, R. B., Selker, H. P., *et al.* "A predictive instrument to improve coronary-care-unit admission practices in acute ischemic heart disease: A prospective multicenter clinical trial." *N. Engl. J. Med.* **310** (1984): 1273–8.

requiring the physicians to use them. Physicians used it in only 2.8 percent of the cases.[7] Low use of well-validated, diagnostic rules by physicians in clinical practice has been noted elsewhere.[8]

The reasons that diagnostic rules are not more widely used are complicated. Physicians, especially in emergency departments, are pressed for time. Pozen's algorithm can be computed in less than 20 seconds, but it requires a preprogrammed hand-held calculator – something most physicians do not carry around with them. Using the worksheet version (if you had one in front of you) it would take you 30–60 seconds to calculate the probability of ischemia. Although this may not seem like a long time, in the emergency department, with many patients in gurneys in front of you, it can seem like an impossibly long task.

Psychological factors also impede the use of diagnostic models by physicians. Medical training has traditionally been akin to apprenticeship. You work with physicians more experienced than yourself until you have enough experience to function on your own. At a certain point, physicians feel that their judgment is accurate (even if studies show that, for some conditions, diagnostic models are more accurate than decisions made by physicians). The physicians in the Corey and Merenstein study complained that they lost confidence in the model when they discovered that two patients with very different characteristics could have the same predicted probability of ischemia. Perhaps, most importantly, as a profession, physicians are not yet comfortable using computer-generated models. But the potential is there. A good diagnostic model can make an intern instantly as good a diagnostician as the head of the department of medicine!

> **TIP**
>
> A good diagnostic algorithm can make an intern as good a diagnostician as the head of the department of medicine!

Before diagnostic models can be used in clinical practice they must be shown to be highly accurate in predicting outcome (Section 12.1). For this reason, developing diagnostic models can be challenging. However, in one respect they are easier to construct than explanatory models. In diagnostic settings, causality is unimportant. For example, diagonal ear lobe creases are associated with coronary events, even with adjustment for known cardiac risk factors including age, left ventricular ejection fraction, cholesterol level, smoking, diabetes, family history, and obesity.[9] No one believes that ear lobe creases cause coronary events. Looked at from a different point of view, lowering a patient's cholesterol level may decrease the risk of a myocardial infarction, but

---

[7] Corey, G. A. and Merenstein, J. H. "Applying the acute ischemic heart disease predictive instrument." *J. Fam. Pract.* **25** (1987): 127–33.

[8] Pearson, S. D., Goldman, L., Garcia, T. B., *et al.* "Physician response to a prediction rule for the triage of emergency department patients with chest pain." *J. Gen. Intern. Med.* **9** (1994): 241–7; Wasson, J. H. and Sox, H. C. "Clinical prediction rules: Have they come of age?" *JAMA* **275** (1996): 641–2; Gehlbach, S. H. "Commentary." *J. Fam. Pract.* **25** (1987): 132–3.

[9] Elliott, W. J. and Powell, L. H. "Diagonal earlobe creases and prognosis in patients with suspected coronary artery disease." *Am. J. Med.* **100** (1996): 205–11.

removing an ear lobe crease with plastic surgery would have no effect on the risk of an infarction. The association of ear lobe creases with coronary events is confounded by some yet-to-be determined cardiac risk factor.

But a patient's ear crease still provides useful clinical information. This is especially true if you are a paramedic evaluating patients with chest pain in the field and have little other information about them. Thus in constructing diagnostic algorithms, we are interested in variables that together accurately predict outcome regardless of whether the effect is confounded by some other variable.

2.5 How is multivariable analysis used in studies of prognosis?

How bad is it, Doc? Will the cancer come back? How long do I have to live? These are some of the most difficult questions clinicians face from their patients. Most ethicists and clinicians agree that patients have a right to an honest answer to these questions. While we will never be able to predict the outcome for any one person, multivariable analysis can provide information on the prognosis of a group of patients with a particular set of known prognostic factors.

For example, Schuchter and colleagues developed a prognostic model using logistic regression for estimating 10-year survival in 488 patients with primary melanoma.[10] They prospectively followed patients with primary melanoma. Ten-year survival was 78 percent. Using multiple logistic regression, they identified four factors associated with survival at ten years (yes/no): age, sex, location (extremity versus axis of body), and lesion thickness. At one extreme, women who were 60 years or younger with a lesion <0.76 mm of thickness on their extremity had an estimated 10-year survival of 99 percent. At the other extreme, men who were older than 60 with a lesion >3.6 mm of thickness on their trunk had an estimated 10-year survival of only 10 percent.

This prognostic model illustrates how different survival can be with the same disease but different patient characteristics. Schuchter and colleagues' model correctly predicted outcome in 74 percent of cases. In other words, if you knew age, sex, location, and lesion thickness, you would correctly predict survival or death at ten years for 74 percent of the sample.

The cynics among you may say: I can do better than that without any prognostic information. If I predict that all patients will be alive at ten years, I will be correct in 78 percent of the cases (10-year survival = 78 percent). This is

---

[10] Schuchter, L., Schultz, D. J., Synnestvedt, M., *et al.* "A prognostic model for predicting a 10-year survival in patients with primary melanoma." *Ann. Intern. Med.* **125** (1996): 369–75.

true, but you would not have correctly predicted any of the deaths. Methods for judging the success of models at predicting dichotomous outcomes are discussed in Section 8.2.B.

Prognostic models provide valid estimates of risk only for patients with similar characteristics to those in the study population. For example, if a prognostic model is based on a sample of males over the age of 50, it will not be helpful in predicting the survival of a 45-year-old woman.

Prognostic models work only when there is a known set of risk factors. They are most useful when they include only those variables readily available to a clinician. If the model requires knowing the genetic markers of the cancer, and testing for those markers is not universally available, the model will be of less help. [11]

Even if all these conditions are met, as is the case with the melanoma study, a model will generally not predict outcome prospectively (with new cases) as well as it does retrospectively (with the cases in the data set from which it was developed). Why? Because the models maximize the correct prediction of the outcome based on the values of the independent and dependent variables in the data set (Section 12.1).

---

[11] For an excellent review of using multivariable models to determine prognosis, see: Braitman, L. E. and Davidoff, F. "Predicting clinical states in individual patients." *Ann. Intern. Med.* **125** (1996): 406–12.

Outcome variables in multivariable analysis

3.1 How does the nature of the outcome variable influence the choice of which type of multivariable analysis to do?

The choice of multivariable analysis depends primarily on the type of outcome variable that you have (Table 3.1). Therefore, I have organized this chapter by outcome variable: interval (Section 3.2), dichotomous (Section 3.3), ordinal (Section 3.4), nominal (Section 3.5), time to occurrence (Sections 3.6–3.9), count (Section 3.10) and incidence rate (Section 3.11). To help orient you, I have included in Table 3.1 examples of each type of outcome variable, and the statistic generally used to perform a bivariate analysis with the same type of data. My hope is that this will ease your transition from performing bivariate analyses to multivariable analyses.

Although different models are used for different outcome variables, it is sometimes possible to change the nature of the outcome variable (or to test more than one form of your outcome variable). Therefore, in Section 3.12, I discuss ways to transform variables so that they can be analyzed using different multivariable techniques.

Each of the multivariable models has a different set of underlying assumptions. Therefore to help you choose the correct model and interpret the output correctly I have included the underlying assumptions for each of the models within each section. In Chapter 9, I review methods of testing the underlying assumption of the multivariable models. Although it may seem artificial to separate the explanation of the assumptions from the testing of them, this distinction mirrors the data analytic process. We choose models that we believe will fit the structure of our data. After we perform the analysis, we check to see if the assumptions of the models are satisfied.

All the models discussed in this chapter assume that each subject has only one value on the outcome variable and that the observations of different subjects are independent. Therefore special methods are needed for longitudinal studies where subjects may be observed repeatedly on the same outcome (e.g.,

Table 3.1 Type of outcome variable determines choice of multivariable analysis.

Type of outcome	Example of outcome variable	Type of bivariate analysis	Type of multivariable analysis
Interval	Blood pressure, weight, temperature	Correlation coefficient, linear regression, *t* test, ANOVA	Multiple linear regression, analysis of variance (and related procedures)
Dichotomous	Death, cancer, intensive care unit admission	Chi-squared, Fisher's exact, *t* test, chi-squared for trend, Mann–Whitney test	Multiple logistic regression
Ordinal	Stage of disease, severity of symptoms	Chi-squared for trend, Mann–Whitney test, Spearman's rank correlation coefficient	Proportional odds regression
Nominal	Cause of death, site of cancer	Chi-squared, ANOVA, Kruskal–Wallis	Multinomial logistic regression
Time to outcome	Time to death, time to cancer	Log-rank	Proportional hazards analysis
Counts	Number of infections, number of hospital admissions	Poisson regression, negative binomial regression	Poisson regression, negative binomial regression
Incidence rates	Rate of new infections, rate of car accidents	z scores	Poisson regression, negative binomial regression

blood pressure at 6 months, blood pressure at 12 months) or for cross-sectional or longitudinal studies where the outcomes of different subjects are correlated (i.e., subjects from the same family will have correlated outcomes). These methods are discussed in Chapter 11.

3.2 What type of multivariable analysis should I use with an interval outcome?

> **DEFINITION**
>
> With an *interval* variable each unit (interval) of change on the scale has an equal quantifiable value.

With an interval variable (also called continuous) each unit (interval) of change on the scale has an equal (numerically) quantifiable value. Examples of interval variables are blood pressure, body weight, and temperature. In these examples, a one-unit change at any point on the scale is equal to a millimeter of mercury, a pound (or kilogram), or a degree, respectively.

If you were performing a bivariate analysis with an interval outcome you would use a *t* test (with a dichotomous independent variable), a correlation

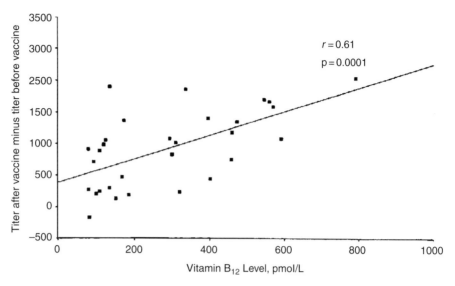

Figure 3.1   Linear association between vitamin B$_{12}$ levels and and the difference between antibody titers before and after pneumococcal vaccination. Reproduced with permission from: Fata, F.T., *et al.* "Impaired antibody responses to pneumococcal polysaccharide in elderly patients with low serum vitamin B$_{12}$ levels." *Ann. Intern. Med.* **124** (1996): 299–304.

coefficient or linear regression (with an interval-independent variable), an analysis of variance (with a nominal independent variable), or Spearman's rank correlation coefficient (with an ordinal or non-normal interval-independent variable) (Table 3.1). Of these techniques only linear regression and analysis of variance can incorporate multiple independent variables; they are discussed below.

3.2.A Multiple linear regression

As implied by the name, multiple linear regression determines the best line for predicting the outcome variable based on the values of the independent variables.

For example, Figure 3.1 shows the relationship between B$_{12}$ levels and the increase in antibody levels following receipt of pneumococcal vaccination among elderly persons.[1] Each square represents an observation (a person),

---

[1] Fata, F.T., Herzlich, B.C., Schiffman, G., *et al.* "Impaired antibody responses to pneumococcal polysaccharide in elderly patients with low serum vitamin B$_{12}$ levels." *Ann. Intern. Med.* **124** (1996): 299–304.

their vitamin B_{12} level (the independent variable), and the increase in their antibody titer after vaccine (the dependent variable). Although arbitrary, the convention is to show the independent variable on the x-axis and the dependent variable on the y-axis.

Least squares linear regression (the most commonly performed method of linear regression) determines the line that minimizes the distance between the data points and the line itself. Although the linear regression line shown in Figure 3.1 may be the best single representation of the data, note that none of the points actually falls on the line and many points are not even that close to the line. Statistical models are, at best, approximations of data. In the case of this data a line is a good, but imperfect representation of the fact that as vitamin B_{12} levels increase, the levels of antibodies also increase from prevaccination levels.

> Least squares linear regression determines the line that minimizes the distance between the data points and the line itself.

The relationship between vitamin B_{12} levels and development of antibodies shown in Figure 3.1 is based on a bivariate analysis. That's the reason the authors perform a simple correlation coefficient ($r = 0.61$) to summarize the relationship. Bivariate statistics may be sufficient if there are no potential confounders of the relationship being studied.

But what if the relationship between B_{12} levels and antibody development is confounded by age? This is a distinct possibility since older persons tend to have lower B_{12} levels and are less likely to respond to vaccinations.

To eliminate confounding by age, the authors adjusted for age, as well as mean corpuscular volume, in a multiple linear regression analysis, adjusting for age. They found that higher vitamin B_{12} levels were significantly associated with greater increases in pneumococcal titers in response to vaccination. Illustrating that multiple analysis is useful not only for eliminating confounding, but also for identifying independent risk factors for an outcome (Section 2.2), the authors found that mean corpuscular volume was also significantly associated with the response to vaccination.

3.2.B Analysis of variance (ANOVA)

Analysis of variance (ANOVA) can also be used to analyze the relationship between multiple independent variables and an outcome variable. The "variance" in the name of the technique refers to the difference between the values of the individual subjects and the mean. The "between-groups" variance is based on the differences between the subjects and the mean of the sample. The "within-groups" variance is based on the differences between the group members and the group mean.

If the means of the groups are very different then the variance calculated, based on the mean of the entire sample (between-groups variance), will be larger than the variance based on the mean of each group (within-groups variance). Assuming there is a large enough sample size, the difference will be statistically significant. If the means of the groups are not very different then the variance calculated, based on the mean of the entire sample, will be similar to the variance calculated based on the mean of each group.

There are several different types of analysis of variance (Table 3.2). The simplest type of ANOVA is a one-way (or one-factor) design in which two or more groups are compared on a single interval variable.[2] For example, we might compare the blood pressure of persons randomized to receive different treatments (e.g., diuretic, beta-blocker, ACE inhibitor). In this case, ANOVA is being used as a bivariate tool not a multivariable one.

ANOVA and related procedures can also be used to answer multivariable questions. For example, a two-way ANOVA can be used to determine the effect of (1) group assignment, (2) other categorical variables (e.g., ethnicity, gender), and (3) the interaction between the assigned group and a categorical variable on an interval outcome. For example, Grande and colleagues used ANOVA to analyze data from a randomized experiment on the impact of drug promotional material.[3] Third- and fourth-year medical students at two schools were randomized to exposure or non-exposure to promotional items for Lipitor® (atorvastatin). One of the schools had a restrictive policy in place limiting pharmaceutical marketing (Penn) and one did not (Miami). The outcome was preference for Lipitor® measured on an interval scale.

The results of the experiment are shown in Figure 3.2. In the top panel you can see that compared to control students, fourth-year students at Miami exposed to Lipitor promotion materials exhibited more favorable attitudes to Lipitor than to Zucar® (simvastatin) a competitor drug. The opposite effect was seen in students at Penn where there was a very restrictive policy concerning drug promotions.

In the second panel, you can see that scores for third-year students, who had not yet formed attitudes towards treatment options, were not affected by the promotion materials. An ANOVA analysis demonstrated that the interaction

---

[2] For a review of analysis of variance see: Katz, M. H. *Study Design and Statistical Analysis: A Practical Guide for Clinicians.* Cambridge: Cambridge University Press, 2006, pp. 88–9; for an excellent free statistical book that includes a thorough discussion of analysis of variance, go to: www.statsoft.com/textbook/stanman.html.

[3] Grande, D., Frosch, D. L., Perkins, A. W., Kahn, B. E. "Effect of exposure to small pharmaceutical promotional items on treatment practices." *Arch. Intern. Med.* **69** (2009): 887–93.

Table 3.2 Analysis of variance techniques.

Types	Indication
Analysis of variance (ANOVA)	Compares two or more groups on an interval outcome. Can incorporate categorical independent variables and the interaction of categorical variables with the main effect.
Analysis of covariance (ANCOVA)	Similar to analysis of variance but can incorporate continuous as well as categorical independent variables in the model.
Multivariate analysis of variance (MANOVA)	Similar to analysis of variance but used when there is more than one dependent variable. Use of MANOVA decreases the chance of making a type I error.
Multivariate analysis of covariance (MANCOVA)	Similar to analysis of covariance but used when there is more than one dependent variable. Use of MANCOVA decreases the chance of making a type I error.
Repeated measures analysis of variance/covariance	Similar to analysis of variance/covariance but can incorporate repeated observations of the same subjects (Section 11.3.D).
Repeated measures multivariate analysis of variance/covariance	Similar to multivariate analysis of variance/covariance but can incorporate repeated observations of the same subjects (Section 11.3.D).

between experimental group and school and class was statistically significant ($P = 0.003$).

In this study the independent variables were categorical (school, class), which are easily incorporated into ANOVA. However, if the independent variables that you need to incorporate are interval (e.g., age, weight) you will need to use analysis of covariance (ANCOVA). With ANCOVA you can incorporate both interval and categorical variables.

For example, in a large multicenter study, diabetics were randomized to receive either continuous glucose monitoring or standard home monitoring.[4] The outcome was a change in the glycated hemoglobin level from baseline to 26 weeks. Because the investigators needed to adjust for both continuous variables (baseline glycated hemoglobin levels) and categorical variables (clinical center) they analyzed their data using ANCOVA. They found that there was a significant interaction between study group and age group. Specifically,

> **DEFINITION**
>
> Analysis of covariance is an extension of analysis of variance that allows incorporation of interval-independent variables.

---

[4] The Juvenile Diabetes Research Foundation Continuous Glucose Monitoring Study Group. "Continuous glucose monitoring and intensive treatment of type 1 diabetes." *N. Engl. J. Med.* **359** (2008): 1464–76.

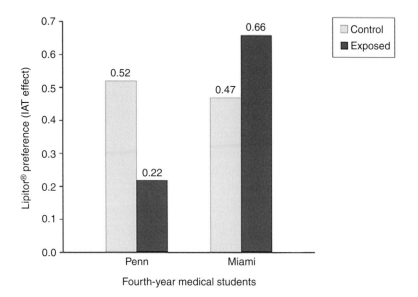

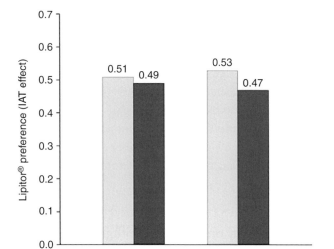

Figure 3.2   Preference for Lipitor® by fourth- and third- year medical students exposed or not exposed to promotional material. Preference is measured using the implicit association test (IAT). Reproduced with permission from Grande, D., *et al.* "Effect of exposure to small pharmaceutical promotional items on treatment practices." *Arch. Intern. Med.* **69** (2009): 887–93.

glycated hemoglobin levels were better among the continuous monitoring group than among the usual care group, but only among subjects greater than 25 years of age. In the other two age groups (8 to 14 years and 15 to 24 years) there was no difference between the glycated levels for the subjects in the two arms of the study. In further analysis, the investigators found that subjects older than 25 years wore the sensors significantly more than younger patients. To the extent that younger patients didn't wear the sensors (which have to be placed subcutaneously and replaced every few days), it is not surprising that the sensors didn't help them to control their glucose levels.

Because of the similarities between analysis of variance and analysis of covariance, your software program may automatically choose which of the two to perform, based on whether or not you enter into the model interval-independent variables.

Multivariate analysis of variance (MANOVA) and multivariate analysis of covariance (MANCOVA) are extensions of analysis of variance and analysis of covariance, respectively, that are used when studying more than one dependent variable. The outcome variables are generally correlated. These procedures are used to decrease the chance of making a type I error (falsely rejecting the null hypothesis).

A MANOVA produces a multivariate F (Wilks' lambda). If the multivariate F test were significant, you would then examine the bivariate F test values. Conversely, if the multivariate F test were not significant you would ignore the individual F tests. Multivariate designs require that the intercorrelations of the outcome variables are homogeneous across the cells of the design.[5]

Adaptations of analysis of variance and analysis of covariance, multivariate analysis of variance and multivariate analysis of covariance, are also available for analyzing repeated observations of the same individuals (Section 11.3.D).

3.2.C Underlying assumptions of multiple linear regression and ANOVA

The underlying assumptions of multiple linear regression and ANOVA are the same (Table 3.3). With both multiple linear regression and ANOVA the outcome can take any positive or negative numeric value, Both techniques assume the outcome has a normal distribution and equal variance around the mean for any value(s) of the independent variable(s).[6] To fulfill this condition your outcome

---

[5] French, A. and Poulsen, J. "Multivariate analysis of variance (MANOVA)." http://online.sfsu.edu/~efc/classes/biol710/manova/manova.htm.

[6] The technical term for equal variance for any value of X is homoscedasticity; "homo" meaning same and "scedastic" from the Greek word "to scatter." For a more detailed explanation of these and the other assumptions of linear regression, see: Kleinbaum, D. G., Kupper, L. L., and Muller, K. E.

Table 3.3 Underlying assumptions of multiple linear regression and analysis of variance.

Type of outcome variable	Interval
Range of values for outcome variable	Any positive or negative number
What is being modeled	Mean
Distribution of outcome variable	Normal
Variance of outcome variable	Equal around the mean

variable should have a bell-shaped curve for any value of your independent variable. This is shown in Figure 3. 3(a). Note that for each of the three values of the independent variable (X_1, X_2, and X_3), the range of values of the dependent variable forms a bell-shaped curve. Equal variance means that the spread of dependent variable values (indicated by arrows) from the mean (indicated with a dotted line) is equal for each value of X. This is the case in Figure 3.3(a).

If you have an interval-independent variable, it is easier to assess these assumptions if you group the independent variable into a few groups. So, for example, in Figure 3.3(a), X_1, X_2, and X_3 may represent a range of values (e.g., age 20–39 years, 40–59 years, 60–79 years).

Figure 3.3(b) shows a bivariate relationship that does not fulfill the assumptions of normal distribution or equal variance. Note that the values of the dependent variable for X_1 and X_2 both produce bell-shaped curves, but the variance is not equal. It is much smaller for values of X_1 than for values of X_2. At X_3 we see a curve with a skewed distribution (long tail). This curve does not have a bell-shaped distribution and the variance is not equal to either of the other two curves. Therefore, the relationship between this independent and dependent variable does not fit the assumptions of normal distribution or equal variance.

Some investigators mistakenly believe that they can evaluate the assumption of normal distribution by assessing only the univariate characteristics of the variable. In other words, they print a histogram for all values of X. If the distribution is bell-shaped they conclude that it fulfills the assumption of normal distribution. However, as explained above, the assumption of normal distribution and equal variance applies to each level of the independent variable, not all values together. Nonetheless, a simple histogram of all your independent variables is a useful first step.

If you find that the univariate distribution of your variable has a significant departure from the bell-shaped curve, it is likely that it will violate the

> Multiple linear regression and ANOVA assume a normal distribution and equal variance around the mean.

Applied Regression Analysis and Other Multivariable Methods (2nd edn). Boston: PWS-Kent, 1988, pp. 44–9.

(a)
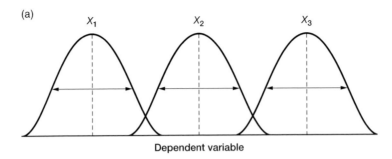

(b)
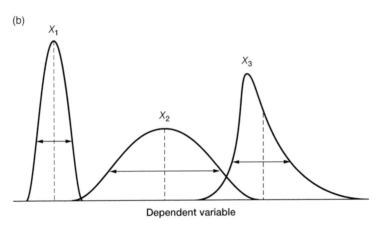

Figure 3.3   Plots of an interval-dependent variable at three different values of the independent variable X. In Figure 3.3(a), the assumptions of normal distribution and equal variance are fulfilled because at all three values of X the curves are bell-shaped and the spread from the mean (indicated by arrows) is equal. In Figure 3.3(b) these assumptions are not met. The assumption of normal distribution is violated because the distribution of values for X_3 does not form a bell-shaped curve. The equal variance assumption is invalid because the spread of values from the mean is different for the three values of X.

assumption of normal distribution and equal variance in bivariate analysis. Since it is easier to review a univariate distribution than a bivariate association, this procedure alerts you to which variables to watch especially carefully in your analysis. In addition to eyeballing the histogram, you can use one of many statistical packages to provide you with a normal probability plot, which should approximate a line if the data are normally distributed. The statistics skewness and kurtosis when high also indicate that the data do not fit a normal distribution, but these are less informative than looking at the histogram.

Besides alerting you to potential violations of the assumptions of normal distribution and equal variance, printing histograms of your dependent and independent variables is a necessary step in cleaning your data. Histograms

TIP

Run histograms for all your variables. They will alert you to: (a) Potential violations of normality and equal variance, (b) implausible values, (c) gaps in your values, and (d) extreme values.

allow you to detect implausible values (e.g., age of 120 years) and help identify gaps in your values. If, for example, you have few observations of persons older than 60 years of age, your results will not necessarily generalize to this older group. Univariate statistics will also help you to detect extreme (but plausible) values (outliers) that might affect your results, such as two octogenarians. If you happen to have two octogenarians and they happen to have extreme values on your outcome variable, they may unduly influence your results (Section 9.5).

Now that you have read all of the above theory and considered what a pain it would be to perform the recommended analysis for each of your independent variables, I am happy to tell you that if your sample size is large (greater than 100), you can assume that the assumption of normal distribution is met (assuming you do not have any unduly influential points). We have the central limit theorem to thank for this great gift,[7] the details of which are beyond the scope of this book.

Only significant departures from equal variance are likely to affect your results. The usual effect would be to decrease the power of your analysis to demonstrate an association between your independent and dependent variables.

If you find *significant* departures from the assumptions of normal distribution and equal variance, and have a small sample, what should you do? You can attempt to transform either the independent or dependent variable so that the relationship fits these assumptions. Commonly performed transformations are the natural logarithm, the square root, the reciprocal, the square, and the arcsine.[8]

Once you have transformed the variable you need to repeat the bivariate relationship to see if indeed the variable more closely fits the assumptions of your model. More sophisticated methods of testing the normality and equal variance are discussed in Section 9.3.

3.2.D Choosing between multiple linear regression and ANOVA

Either technique will yield the same answer, assuming you set up the models in similar ways. Assuming you have more than two groups, to analyze the data using multiple linear regression you will need to create multiple dichotomous variables to represent the groups (see Section 4.2).

> **TIP**
>
> If your sample size is large (greater than 100), you can assume that the assumption of normality is met.

> **TIP**
>
> If you find significant departures from the assumptions of normality and equal variance try transforming the independent or dependent variable.

> **TIP**
>
> Multiple linear regression and ANOVA will yield the same answer if you set up the models in similar ways.

---

[7] For more on the central limit theorem see: Rosner, B. *Fundamentals of Biostatistics* (5th edn). Pacific Grove: Doxbury, 2000, pp. 174–6.

[8] For a fuller discussion of these transformations see: Kleinbaum, D. G., Kupper, L. L., and Muller, K. E. *Applied Regression Analysis and Other Multivariable Methods* (2nd edn). Boston: PWS-Kent, 1988, pp. 220–1.

In general, multiple linear regression is more commonly used with observational data, and analysis of variance is more commonly used with experimental designs. Multiple linear regression is more commonly used in the medical literature, and analysis of variance is more commonly used in the behavioral literature.

3.3 What type of multivariable analysis should I use with a dichotomous outcome?

A dichotomous variable (the simplest kind of categorical variable) has two discrete values (categories) at a discrete point in time, for example: alive or dead; development of cancer: yes or no.

For bivariate analyses of dichotomous outcomes we use chi-squared and Fisher's exact test with dichotomous and nominal independent variables, t test with interval-independent variables, and chi-squared for trend and Mann–Whitney test with ordinal and non-normal interval-independent variables (Table 3.1). But these statistics cannot be used if there is more than one independent variable. To perform multivariable analysis with dichotomous outcomes use multiple (binary) logistic regression.[9]

To appreciate the value of logistic regression for analyzing dichotomous variables, look at Figure 3.4. It shows the association between skeletal muscle strength (measured in the deltoid muscle) and presence of cardiomyopathy among alcoholics.[10] You can see that at low levels of muscle strength (left-hand side of the curve), there are several closed circles (representing patients with cardiomyopathy) while there are no open circles (patients with normal cardiac function). In contrast, at high levels of muscle strength (right-hand side of the curve) there are many open circles and few closed circles, reflecting that patients without cardiomyopathy have normal muscle strength. The triangles indicate the probability of cardiomyopathy at different levels of muscle strength. The curve connecting the triangles shows that at intermediate levels of muscle strength, there is a rapidly decreasing proportion of patients with cardiomyopathy as muscle strength increases.

The probability of cardiomyopathy, as with any event, cannot be less than zero or greater than one. The value of logistic regression is that it incorporates this assumption (Table 3.4). Logistic regression models the "logit" of the

> **DEFINITION**
>
> A *dichotomous* variable has two discrete values.

---

[9] Generally people simply refer to this technique as multiple logistic regression or logistic regression. I have used the binary here, and in other places, to help distinguish it from the related ordinal logistic regression and multinomial (polytomous) logistic regression.

[10] Fernandez-Sola, J., Estruch, R., Grau, J. M., *et al.* "The relationship of alcoholic myopathy to cardiomyopathy." *Ann. Intern. Med.* **120** (1994): 529–36.

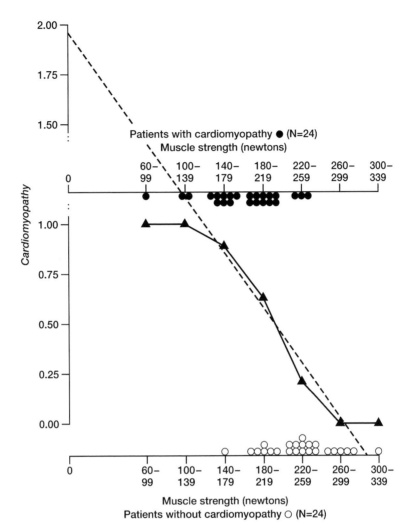

Figure 3.4   Z-shaped association between skeletal muscle strength and presence of cardiomyopathy among alcoholics. The closed circles are patients with cardiomyopathy and the open circles are patients without cardiomyopathy. The triangles show the observed proportion of patients with cardiomyopathy at different levels of muscle strength. Data are from Fernandez-Sola, J., Estruch, R., Grau, J.M., *et al.* "The relationship of alcoholic myopathy to cardiomyopathy." *Ann. Intern. Med.* **120** (1994): 529–36.

outcome. The logit is the natural logarithm of the odds of the outcome. The odds of the outcome is the probability of having the outcome divided by the probability of not having the outcome. Whereas the logit can take on any value from minus to plus infinity, the probability, which is the inverse of the logit, can only take on values of zero to one. This gives the logistic function an S or

Table 3.4 Underlying assumptions of logistic regression.

Type of outcome variable	Dichotomous
Range of values for outcome variable	0 to 1
What is being modeled?	The logarithm of the odds of the outcome (referred to as logit)
Distribution of outcome variable	Binomial
Variance of outcome variable	Depends only on the mean

Z shape (depending on which way the outcome variable is configured). As you can see in Figure 3.4, this shape fits the data. Note that as the probability of outcome approaches zero or one, further increases or decreases in the independent variable have little effect on the outcome.

I have drawn a linear regression line (the dotted line) so that you can appreciate that a linear function would not be as good a model for the data. Cardiomyopathy is either present or not. Yet the line would predict that a patient with muscle strength of less than 100 newtons would have a value greater than one on the cardiomyopathy variable. The line would also indicate that a patient with muscle strength of 300 newtons or greater would have a negative value on the cardiomyopathy variable. Obviously, these values are impossible.

Although this S- or Z-shaped function is useful, remember that it is still just a model. The curve I have drawn in Figure 3.4 is based on the actual data. The estimated curve would be of a similar shape but would not go exactly through the boxes. We will take up the issue of how to assess how well a model fits the observed data in Section 8.2.

With logistic regression, the dependent variable is assumed to have a binomial distribution. A binomial distribution describes the number of successes or failures (e.g., yes or no; survival or death) in a series of *independent* trials. Independent trials mean that the outcome for one subject is independent of the outcome for another subject. In other words, the outcomes are not clustered owing to being from the same individuals, families, or medical practices. There are methods for dealing with clustered effects (Chapter 11). The variances in logistic regression are assumed to depend only on the mean.

The model in Figure 3.4 illustrates the bivariate relationship between skeletal muscle strength and cardiomyopathy. However, the value of multiple logistic regression analysis compared to bivariate techniques is that the former can assess the relationship of an independent variable to a dichotomous outcome with adjustment for other factors.

For example, logistic regression was used to demonstrate that cardiopulmonary resuscitation (CPR) might be effective with just chest compressions and no rescue breathing. The reason that this is important is that some bystanders do not perform CPR because of concern about transmission of disease with mouth-to-mouth rescue breathing. Others find CPR with both cardiac compressions and rescue breathing to be too complicated to learn. If CPR with only chest compressions were as good as CPR with both chest compressions and rescue breathing, public education campaigns should focus on chest compressions.

This question was studied in Japan by having paramedics record whether patients with bystander-witnessed cardiac arrest were receiving bystander CPR and if so of which kind.[11] The investigators compared persons who received chest compressions only to those who received both chest compressions and rescue breathing. Although the difference is not statistically significant, the percentage of persons having a favorable neurologic outcome is actually higher in the group of persons who received only chest compressions. However, this result could be confounded because there were statistically significant differences between the two groups. In particular, persons who received CPR with chest compressions only were more likely to be male, to experience their arrest at home, and to have their CPR performed by laypersons. Perhaps one of these differences explains the better outcomes?

As you can see from Table 3.5, this is not the case. Using multiple logistic regression to adjust for male sex, where the arrest occurred, as well as who performed the arrests, the investigators found that the effect actually got stronger:[12] persons who received only chest compressions were statistically more likely to have a positive neurologic outcome (95% confidence intervals exclude 1.0). If it seems to you impossible that CPR that has only chest compressions could be superior to CPR with both, consider that if there is only one bystander performing CPR, time spent doing respirations takes time away from compressions, which may be more valuable. Despite this being an observational study, an accompanying editorial recommended changing the CPR guidelines to compressions only for cardiac arrests.[13]

3.4 What type of multivariable analysis should I use with an ordinal variable?

An ordinal variable (also known as a ranked variable) has multiple categories that can be ordered or ranked. For example, the New York Heart Association's functional classification of cardiac function is an ordinal scale with four levels.

---

[11] Sos-Kanto Study Group. "Cardiopulmonary resuscitation by bystanders with chest compression only (SOS-Kanto): an observational study." Lancet **369** (2007): 920–6.

[12] As the effect became stronger with statistical adjustment this is an example of a suppressor effect (Section 1.3).

[13] Ewy, G. A. "Cardiac arrest – guideline changes urgently needed." Lancet **369** (2009): 882–4.

Table 3.5 Compressions-only versus conventional CPR in producing a good neurologic outcome.

	Compressions-only Good neurologic outcome N (%)	Conventional CPR Good neurologic outcome N (%)	Bivariate odds ratio (95% CI)	Multivariable odds ratio (95% CI)
Yes	27 (6%)	30 (4%)	1.5 (0.9–2.5)	2.2 (1.2–4.2)
No	412 (94%)	682 (96%)		
	Chi-squared P value = 0.14			

Although the levels can be ordered, there is not a numerically quantifiable difference between level I (no limit in physical activity) and level II (slight limitation in physical activity). The difference between level I and II is not equal to the difference between level III (marked limitation of physical activity) and level IV (inability to carry out any physical activity without discomfort).

For bivariate analysis of ordinal outcomes, we use chi-squared for trend and Mann–Whitney test with dichotomous independent variables, Kruskal–Wallis test with nominal independent variables, and Spearman's rank correlation coefficient with interval and ordinal independent variables (see Table 3.1). However, none of these procedures can incorporate multiple independent variables.

To perform multivariable analysis with ordinal outcomes use an adaptation of logistic regression: proportional odds regression.[14] Proportional odds regression (also referred to as ordinal logistic, ordered logistic regression, ordered logit, cumulative odds models, or constrained cumulative logit model) models the cumulative logit across the categories of an ordinal outcome (Table 3.6).

Proportional odds regression assesses the relationship between the independent variables and the ordinal variable at all possible cut-points of the ordinal outcome. For example, in a 5-level ordinal outcome, there are 4 possible cut-points: 1 vs. 2–5, 1–2 vs. 3–5, 1–3 vs. 4–5, and 1–4 vs. 5 (there is one cut-point less than the number of categories). If we were to use multiple logistic regression to calculate a logit for each of these cut-offs, we would have 4 logits, representing the log odds of the outcome at each cut-off. With proportional odds regression we can estimate one logit, a "cumulative" or "average" of the logits for the different cut-points. The advantage of this approach is that we then have one estimate of the impact of each independent variable on the outcome, rather than four different estimates corresponding to the four different cut-points.

> **DEFINITION**
>
> An *ordinal* variable has multiple categories that can be ordered.

> Use proportional odds regression with ordinal outcomes.

> Proportional odds regression calculates an "average" of the logits that would be obtained if you calculated separate logits at each of the possible cut-points of the outcome variable.

---

[14] See: Scott, S.C., Goldberg, M.S., and Mayo, N.E. "Statistical assessment of ordinal outcomes in comparative studies." *J. Clin. Epidemiol.* **50** (1997): 45–55; Menard, S. *Applied Logistic Regression Analysis.* Thousand Oaks, CA: Sage Publications, 1995, pp. 80–90.

Table 3.6 Underlying assumptions of proportional odds logistic regression.

Type of outcome variable	Ordinal
Range of values for outcome variable	Number of categories
What is being modeled	The cumulative logit
Odds ratios at different cut-offs of the outcome variable	Homogeneous

For example, Hylek and colleagues used proportional odds regression to identify independent predictors of the severity of stroke in patients with non-valvular atrial fibrillation.[15] Seriousness of stroke was ranked in three ordered levels:

1. Minor stroke: no neurologic sequelae or a deficit that did not interfere with independent living.
2. Major stroke: neurologic impairment preventing independent living.
3. Severe stroke: hospital death or total dependence after hospital discharge.

Since there are three levels, there are two possible cut-points: 1 versus 2 and 3 (minor stroke versus major and severe stroke); 1 and 2 versus 3 (minor and major versus severe stroke).

Table 3.7 shows the odds ratios for the association between a number of different independent variables and the severity of the stroke. Patients with heart failure, older patients, and patients who received no therapy or warfarin at a nontherapeutic dose were significantly likelier to have a more serious stroke. These odds ratios are adjusted for all of the other variables shown in the table. This study is important because it shows that even when anticoagulation doesn't prevent a stroke, it appears to lessen the severity.

Because there is only one odds ratio for each independent variable even though there are two possible odds ratios that could be calculated at the different cut-points, you will immediately appreciate that for the odds ratio to be meaningful it must be about the same at the different possible cut-points. This is referred to as the proportional odds assumption.

For example, the odds ratio for the association between no antithrombotic therapy and severity of stroke is 2.2 (Table 3.7), indicating that not being on therapy increases the risk of having a more harmful stroke. But what if this "average" odds ratio is not a good representation of the two odds ratios

TIP

The proportional odds assumption means that the result is about the same regardless of the cut-point of the ordinal variable.

---

[15] Hylek, E. M., Go, A. S., Chang, Y. "Effect of intensity of oral anticoagulation on stroke severity and mortality in atrial fibrillation." *N. Engl. J. Med.* **349** (2003): 1019–26.

Table 3.7 Independent predictors of the severity of ischemic stroke in patients with nonvalvular atrial fibrillation.

Risk factor	Odds ratio (95% CI)	P value
Heart failure	1.6 (1.1–2.2)	0.009
Age (per decade)	1.5 (1.2–1.8)	<0.001
Antithrombotic medication at admission		
None	2.2 (1.3–3.8)	0.004
Aspirin	1.3 (0.7–2.3)	0.40
Warfarin, nontherapeutic dose	1.9 (1.1–3.4)	0.03
Warfarin, therapeutic dose	1.0 (reference)	–
Female sex	1.1 (0.8–1.5)	0.54
Coronary heart disease	1.1 (0.8–1.5)	0.59
Diabetes mellitus	1.3 (0.9–1.9)	0.18
Hypertension	1.2 (0.9–1.7)	0.24
Prior ischemic stroke	1.1 (0.8–1.5)	0.71

Data from Hylek, E. M., *et al.* "Effect of intensity of oral anticoagulation on stroke severity and mortality in atrial fibrillation." *N. Engl. J. Med.* **349** (2003): 1019–26.

representing the two possible cut-offs? What if the odds ratio is 1.0 for the association between no antithrombotic therapy and minor stroke versus major and severe stroke, but 4.0 for the association between minor and major versus severe stroke? In this case the "average" odds ratio of 2.2 from the proportional odds model does not capture the true relationship between antithrombotic therapy and severity of stroke at all cut-points of severity.

To assess the validity of the proportional odds assumption use the score test. It is discussed in Section 9.8.

3.5 What type of multivariable analysis should I use with a nominal outcome?

A nominal variable has multiple categories that cannot be ordered. For example, there is no sensible numeric ordering of cause of death or type of cancer. In your database you may have assigned numbers to represent the different categories of a nominal variable (e.g., 1 = breast cancer, 2 = colon cancer, 3 = lung cancer, etc.) but the numbers are purely symbols and have no numeric meaning. The mean and the median are equally meaningless, if you make the mistake of calculating them.

Use multinomial logistic regression with nominal outcomes.

For bivariate analyses of nominal outcomes we use chi-squared analyses for dichotomous and nominal independent variables, ANOVA for

Table 3.8 Underlying assumptions of multinomial logistic regression.

Type of outcome variable	Nominal
Range of values for outcome variable	Number of categories; one category must serve as the reference category
What is being modeled	The logit (compared to the reference category)

interval-independent variables, and Kruskal–Wallis test for ordinal and non-normal interval-independent variables (Table 3.1).

When you need to analyze a nominal outcome and adjust for multiple independent variables, use multinomial logistic regression (also referred to as polytomous logistic regression) (Table 3.8).[16]

With multinomial logistic regression, one of the categories is designated (by the investigator) to be the reference category. The choice of reference category does not affect the mathematical answer, but it does affect how the results are reported. Choose for your reference category either the largest category or the one to which you wish to draw contrast.

In a multinomial logistic regression, the model compares each of the categories of the outcome variable to the reference category for each of the independent variables. The number of comparisons is equal to one minus the number of categories of the outcome variable. If there are four categories, A, B, C and D, and the reference category is A, a multinomial logistic regression will calculate the logit for being in category B versus A, category C versus A, and category D versus A. Of note, it will not calculate the logit for being in category B versus C, or C versus D.

For example, Murphy and colleagues were interested to see whether there had been improvement over time in the inclusion of ethnic minorities in clinical cancer trials.[17] Since ethnicity is a nominal outcome, they used multinomial logistic regression to determine the impact of calendar year (independent variable) on ethnic composition of subjects (outcome), with adjustment for age, sex, and cancer type. As you can see in Table 3.9, participants enrolled in 2000–2002 were less likely to be African-American (compared to whites – the reference group) than persons enrolled in 1996–1998; in other words, there was less inclusion of African-Americans. There were no significant changes over time among the other ethnic populations compared to Caucasians.

> **TIP**
>
> Multinomial logistic regression requires choosing a reference category: choose either the largest category or the one to which you wish to draw contrast to.

---

[16] Multinomial means more than two categories, so actually proportional odds regression (Section 3.4) is a special type of multinomial logistic regression. But usually the term multinomial logistic regression refers to a logistic model with a nominal outcome.

[17] Murphy, V. H., Krumholz, H. M., Gross, C. P. "Participation in cancer clinical trials: race-, sex-, and age-based disparities." *JAMA* **291** (2004): 2720–6.

Table 3.9 Changes in enrollment of ethnic minorities over time, 2000–2002 vs. 1996–1998.

Group	Enrollment of ethnic minorities vs. Caucasians, 2000–2002 vs. 1996–1998	
	Relative risk ratio* (95% CI)	*P* value
Caucasian	1.0 (Referent)	
Hispanic	0.88 (0.72–1.08)	0.023
African-American	0.76 (0.65–0.89)	<0.001
Asian/Pacific Islander	0.99 (0.83–1.18)	0.91
American Indian/Alaskan Native	0.80 (0.57–1.10)	0.17

* Adjusted for age, sex, and cancer type using multinomial logistic regression.
 Data from Murphy, V. H., *et al.* "Participation in cancer clinical trials: race-, sex-, and age-based disparities." *JAMA* **291** (2004): 2720–6.

    Considering the relative risk ratios for each ethnic category you may realize that you could estimate a similar risk ratio by performing four different logistic regression analyses (five categories equal four models); in each analysis you would include only the subjects in one of the categories (e.g., African-Americans) and those in the reference group (e.g., Caucasians). Indeed, if you were to do this, the relative risk you would obtain from each logistic regression model would likely be similar to the estimates produced by the multinomial logistic regression model.[18] The difference is that with the individual logistic regression models the relationship of the independent variables to the outcome would be based on the separate samples, while with multinomial logistic regression, the relationship of the independent variables to the outcome would be based on the entire sample. Because each of the categories is compared to a reference group, there is no proportional odds assumption with multinomial logistic regression.

3.6 What type of multivariable analysis should I use with a time-to-outcome variable?

Time-to-outcome refers to the study of events – such as death or development of cancer – that occur over a period of time (e.g., five years) (Table 3.1). For bivariate analysis of time-to-outcome variables we draw a Kaplan–Meier curve

---

[18] For an illustration see: Hosmer D. W., and Lemeshow, S. *Applied Logistic Regression.* (2nd edn) New York, NY: Wiley, 2000, p. 279–80.

Table 3.10 Underlying assumptions of proportional hazards regression.

Type of outcome variable	Time to outcome
Range of values for outcome variable	0 or 1; time from point 0
What is being modeled	The logarithm of the relative hazard
Censored observations	Censored cases have the same rate of outcome as noncensored cases
Relative hazards over time	Proportional

for each group and compare the curves using log-rank statistics. However, log-rank statistics cannot incorporate multiple independent variables.

When you need to perform multivariable analysis with time-to-outcome data, use proportional hazards analysis (Table 3.10). For example, Hannan and colleagues compared time to death for patients who received drug-eluting stents to those who received coronary artery bypass grafting (CABG).[19] For patients with three-vessel disease the survival of those who received CABG and those who received drug-eluting stents was almost identical (at 18 months 93.4% vs. 93.7%) (Figure 3.5). However, patients were not randomized to receive CABG versus a drug-eluting stent. In general, patients who receive CABG were older, had more cardiac disease, and more comorbid conditions. When the authors used proportional hazards analysis to adjust for potential confounders, including age, ejection fracture, prior myocardial infarction, and comorbid disease, they found that CABG was associated with a significantly lower rate of death (relative hazard = 0.80; 95% CI 0.65–0.97).

> Proportional hazards analysis can incorporate subjects with differing lengths of follow-up.

Proportional hazards analysis, unlike the other multivariable techniques discussed thus far in this chapter, enables you to incorporate subjects with differing lengths of follow-up in your analysis. Differing lengths of follow-up occur commonly in longitudinal studies for a variety of reasons. Subjects may decide they no longer wish to participate. They may move. They may die. They may have to be withdrawn owing to a side effect they have developed. Sometimes you will not know why a person is lost to follow-up; they just are.

> **TIP**
>
> Time-to-outcome models allow inclusion of subjects with differing lengths of follow-up.

Coping with subjects who do not finish a study is one major way in which clinical research is different from other types of research. In laboratory research, it is usually possible to control conditions (e.g., laboratory animals, cell cultures) so that no observations are lost. Much of social science research (and some clinical research) is conducted using cross-sectional designs (surveying people about independent variables and outcomes at the same time). Thus while there

---

[19] Hannan, E. L. Wu, C., Walford, G. *et al.* "Drug-eluting stents vs. coronary-artery bypass grafting in multivessel coronary disease." *N. Engl. J. Med.* **358** (2008): 331–41.

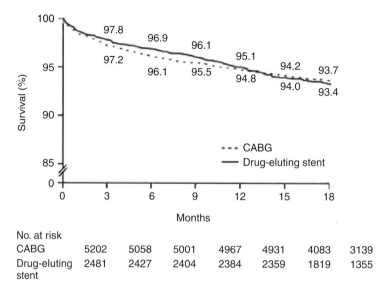

are always people who choose not to participate, subjects are not lost during the study. However, for longitudinal studies (studies of people over time) subjects are invariably lost. For example, if you look at the legend under Figure 3.5 from the study of CABG vs. drug-eluting stents, you will note that there are only 3139 CABG patients at risk for death at 18 months, even though there were 5202 patients at the start of the observation period. This is a decrease of 39% of the sample, even though only 6.3% of patients died.

One method of dealing with such subjects is to delete them. Indeed, if you are using a simple cumulative outcome at a particular point in time (e.g., death at three years: yes or no) you have no choice but to drop subjects who leave the study prior to completion. If the investigators of the CABG vs. drug-eluting stents had chosen this method, they would have to have deleted all subjects who were not available for observation at 18 months and were not known to be dead. Omitting subjects decreases the power of a study and potentially introduces bias.

What we would ideally like is a technique that allows subjects to contribute information until they leave the study. Such a technique exists. It is called censoring and it is a major element of all types of survival analysis, including proportional hazards analysis, which was the technique that was used to adjust for confounders in the analysis of CABG vs. drug-eluting stents.

Besides allowing us to incorporate subjects who are lost to follow-up, censoring has broader implications. It allows us to analyze, within one study, subjects with unequal lengths of follow-up for a variety of reasons (Table 3.11). Indeed, all subjects in a proportional hazards analysis who do not experience the outcome of interest are censored, if not during the course of the study, then at the end of the study.

The underlying assumption of censoring is that if subjects could be followed beyond the point in time when they are censored, they would have the same rate of outcome as those not censored at that time. Another way of saying this is that the censoring occurs randomly, independent of outcome.

To understand the assumptions of censoring, let's look at the Kaplan–Meier survival graph of 100 persons shown in Figure 3.6. The tick marks on the survival function show where persons are censored – that is, where they leave the analysis. Under the *x*-axis of Figure 3.6, I have shown the number of persons who are at risk for outcome (i.e., have not yet experienced the outcome and have not been censored) and the percent survival.

At time 0, everyone is alive and we have 100% survival. As time passes, people die and percent survival decreases. At two years, survival is 86%. Does this mean that 14 participants died and 86 are still alive? No. In fact, there were only 10 deaths.

When you have censoring, the probability of surviving to the end of the follow-up period is not simply the proportion of the original sample known to be alive at the end of the study. The censored subjects contribute information until the time that they leave the analysis. To account for this, we compute a current event rate based on the number of subjects alive and not censored at each point that an event occurs. These current event rates can then be used to compute cumulative survival at the end of the study period (in this case two years). Here's how: Survival to the end is equivalent to surviving each moment in the entire period. We can write the probability of surviving each moment as a product: the product of surviving the first moment times the conditional probability of surviving the second, given that you survived the first, times the conditional probability of surviving the third, given that you survived the first two, and so on, through the last moment. In turn, we can estimate each of these conditional probabilities as one minus the current event rate.

TIP

Censoring allows subjects to contribute information until they leave the study.

DEFINITION

Censoring is used to incorporate subjects with differing lengths of follow-up for a variety of reasons.

Censoring assumes that if subjects could be followed beyond the censor date, they would have the same rate of outcome as those not censored at that time.

Table 3.11 Reasons for censoring observations.

Reason for censoring	Examples
1 Lost to follow-up.	Subject moves, doesn't wish to participate, stops attending a particular clinic.
2 Subject has an outcome that precludes the study outcome (also known as alternative outcomes or competing risks).	Death from coronary artery disease in a study of cancer incidence.
3 Subject is withdrawn from study.	Development of side effects, not ethical to continue treatment or placebo.
4 Varying dates of enrollment.	Study enrolls subjects over a two-year period.
5 End of study.	All subjects who have not experienced outcome are considered censored at the end of the study.

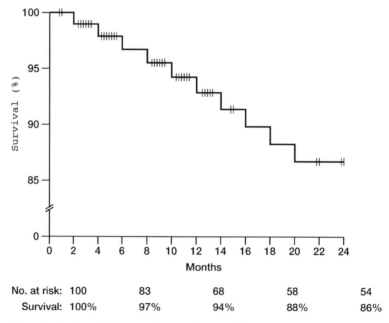

No. at risk:	100	83	68	58	54
Survival:	100%	97%	94%	88%	86%

Figure 3.6   Hypothetical survival experience of 100 subjects.

The cumulative survival at a particular time is simply the conditional probability for that time multiplied by the conditional probability for the prior time at which an event occurred. Because the conditional probabilities are multiplied, this method is sometimes referred to as the product-limit method. For all moments when no event occurs (such as at 3 months in Figure 3.6 and Table 3.12 when there are six censored subjects but no outcome events), the

Table 3.12 Calculation of cumulative survival.

Study time (months)	No. of subjects at risk for outcome	No. of outcomes	No. censored	Current event rate (no. outcomes/ no. subjects at risk)	Conditional probability (1– current event rate)	Cumulative survival
1	100	0	2	0/100 = 0	1 – 0 = 1	1
2	98	1	0	1/98 = 0.01	1 – 0.01 = 0.99	(1)(0.99) = 0.99
3	97	0	6	0/97 = 0	1 – 0 = 1	(0.99)(1) = 0.99
4	91	1	0	1/91 = 0.01	1 – 0.01 = 0.99	(0.99)(0.99) = 0.98
5	90	0	7	0/90 = 0	1 – 0 = 1	(0.98)(1) = 0.98
6	83	1	0	1/83 = 0.01	1 – 0.01 = 0.99	(0.98)(0.99) = 0.97
8	82	1	0	1/82 = 0.01	1 – 0.01 = 0.99	(0.97)(0.99) = 0.96
9	81	0	6	0/81 = 0	1 – 0 = 1	(0.96)(1) = 0.96
10	75	1	0	1/75 = 0.01	1 – 0.01 = 0.99	(0.96)(0.99) = 0.95
11	74	0	6	0/74 = 0	1 – 0 = 1	(0.95)(1) = 0.95
12	68	1	0	1/68 = 0.01	1 – 0.01 = 0.99	(0.95)(0.99) = 0.94
13	67	0	5	0/67 = 0	1 – 0 = 1	(0.94)(1) = 0.94
14	62	1	0	1/62 = 0.02	1 – 0.02 = 0.98	(0.94)(0.98) = 0.92
15	61	0	2	0/61 = 0	1 – 0 = 1	(0.92)(1) = 0.92
16	59	1	0	1/59 = 0.02	1 – 0.02 = 0.98	(0.92)(0.98) = 0.90
18	58	1	0	1/58 = 0.02	1 – 0.02 = 0.98	(0.90)(0.98) = 0.88
20	57	1	0	1/57 = 0.02	1 – 0.02 = 0.98	(0.88)(0.98) = 0.86
22	56	0	2	0/56 = 0	1 – 0 = 1	(0.86)(1) = 0.86
24	54	0	2	0/54 = 0	1 – 0 = 1	(0.86)(1) = 0.86

conditional probability is one, and so it doesn't change the product. These calculations are illustrated in Table 3.12.

Note that censored observations contribute to the analysis until they leave the study, with the provision that they must be in the study at the time that at least one outcome event occurs. Looked at from a different perspective, if observations are censored before any events occur, as is the case with the two censored observations that occur in this example at 1 month, the censored observations would not contribute to the analysis at all (because to be included in the denominator of the current event rate they must still be in the study when the outcome occurs).

What does survival analysis assume about those persons who are censored? It assumes that their rate of outcome is no higher or lower than subjects who stay in the analysis at that point. So if all subjects could be followed to two years in my hypothetical example, how many would have died? The answer is 14. Why? Because if no one were censored then at two years we would have the full sample size of 100. To yield a survival rate of 86%, 14 persons would have died.

I'm sure you can appreciate that this is not a trivial assumption you are making about censored observations. After all, you cannot prove that censored observations have the same rate of outcome as those that are uncensored. If you actually knew the time to outcome for the censored observations they wouldn't need to be censored! What you as an investigator must address is the likelihood that the censoring assumption is valid based on your understanding of why people have been censored (Section 3.7).

Although I have put tick marks on the survival curve and put the number of subjects at risk for outcome under the graph, most published studies will show you one or the other. The number of persons at risk decreases as persons are censored or experience the outcome. This can be seen in Figure 3.5 from the study of CABG vs. drug-eluting stents.

Sometimes published survival curves do not show either ticks for censored observations or the number of subjects at risk as the study progresses. This is a serious limitation because without this information you cannot assess how much the sample is shrinking as the study progresses. As the sample size shrinks, the data no longer represent the survival experience of the full sample. One tip-off that the sample size is shrinking is large "steps" at the end of the curve. As the sample size decreases, the steps of the curve become larger, because an outcome makes a larger difference in the proportion surviving. This is illustrated in Figure 3.6 and Table 3.12. (Note in the table that a single outcome occurring at the end of the study has a larger current event rate than an outcome occurring earlier on in the study.)

3.7 How likely is it that the censoring assumption is valid in my study?

The likelihood that the censoring assumption is valid depends a great deal on the reason for the censored observations.

3.7.A Loss to follow-up

Subjects may be lost to follow-up because they have grown weary of participating in a study (especially if it involves frequent office visits and blood draws). For this reason, many longitudinal studies go to great effort to keep subjects involved, including providing stipends for each visit with a bonus for completing the study, newsletters to keep subjects informed about the progress of the study, and socials to enhance the cohesion of participants.

In the case of retrospective medical record review studies, subjects will be lost to follow-up and you will not know why. You will know only that after a certain period of time there are no further entries in the chart.

Of all reasons for censoring, losses to follow-up are the most problematic for meeting the censoring assumptions.

Of all reasons for censoring, losses to follow-up are the most problematic for meeting the censoring assumptions. Since the participants are lost, you are unlikely to know what has happened to them after leaving the study. For this reason, it may be problematic to assume that the rate of outcome for the censored observations is the same as that for the uncensored subjects. Also, several studies have found that persons who drop out of studies are different from those who remain in the study. For example, a randomized controlled trial of zidovudine in HIV-infected persons found that persons who were lost to follow-up were more likely to have deteriorating immune function during the trial than those who remained in the trial.[20] (They probably left the trial because they knew they were not doing well and wanted to seek other treatment.)

3.7.B Alternative outcome

Some of your subjects may need to be censored because they experience an outcome that precludes the outcome of interest in your study. This is often referred to as competing risks. For example, consider a study that randomized persons with atrial fibrillation to warfarin or to the standard treatment at that time (aspirin or no treatment at all).[21] Stroke was the outcome of interest. The investigators therefore censored persons who died from causes other than stroke (e.g., cardiac events, cancer).

Although it is common to censor persons who have an alternative outcome that precludes the outcome of interest, most studies with a main outcome other than death will also report the results for death as an outcome. There are several reasons for this. Even if warfarin prevents stroke in patients with atrial fibrillation as shown in this study, if subjects treated with warfarin do not also live longer, the therapy may not be as strongly recommended. Knowing that the rate of stroke was lower but the rate of death was higher certainly would sway your view of warfarin as a treatment. This could happen if the treatment was effective against stroke but had a life-threatening side effect (such as bleeds in the case of warfarin).

Another reason to include death as an outcome is that there may be some question as to whether an alternative outcome truly excludes the outcome of interest. Even events that appear unrelated to the outcome of interest may be related. In the context of the atrial fibrillation study, consider someone who

---

[20] Volberding, P. A., Lagakos, S. W., Koch, M. A., *et al*. "Zidovudine in asymptomatic human immunodeficiency virus infection: A controlled trial in persons with fewer than 500 CD4-positive cells per cubic millimeter." *N. Engl. J. Med.* **322** (1990): 941–9.

[21] The Boston Area Anticoagulation Trial for Atrial Fibrillation Investigators. "The effect of low-dose warfarin on the risk of stroke in patients with nonrheumatic atrial fibrillation." *N. Engl. J. Med.* **323** (1990): 1505–11.

died in a car accident. Could you be certain that they did not have a stroke while behind the wheel?

To minimize bias in determining whether an outcome is truly unrelated to the outcome of interest, a study should have objective a-priori criteria as to what constitutes an alternative outcome. In addition, a review committee that is masked to the treatment assignment should make judgments on individual cases. This is exactly what was done in the study of warfarin in patients with atrial fibrillation.

However, even with the best criteria and objective reviewers, you may mistakenly assume that some outcomes are unrelated to your outcome of interest when, perhaps, they are related. In the atrial fibrillation study there were 37 deaths; only one was caused by stroke. The warfarin group had a lower rate of death overall, a lower rate of death owing to cardiac causes, and a lower rate of death owing to noncardiac causes. Since warfarin was not anticipated to have any effect on mortality other than decreasing deaths caused by stroke, these findings suggest two possibilities. Warfarin may prevent death owing to other causes, or some of the deaths attributed to other causes may have actually been caused by unrecognized strokes. The possibility of unrecognized strokes does not weaken the findings. If there were missed strokes in the non-warfarin group it would only strengthen the treatment effect of warfarin. But for the purposes of this discussion, I think this is a good example of how hard it is to correctly categorize nonoutcome-related events.

When death is a common alternative outcome, as it is in any long-term study of elderly or very ill people, competing mortality may bias your estimates of time to outcome. This will occur if the likelihood of outcome would have been higher in those persons who died had they not died. The bias of competing risks can be avoided by not using outcomes other than death (since no outcome precludes death). But in many cases we are interested in these other outcomes. A reasonable compromise is to report both (as was done in the atrial fibrillation trial). More sophisticated methods for dealing with competing risks are beyond the scope of this book.[22]

3.7.C Withdrawal

Persons may withdraw from a study because they do not think the treatment is helping, because they want to receive a treatment and believe they were randomized to placebo, because they have a side effect, or because they find the

---

[22] Pepe, M. S., Longton, G., Pettinger, M., *et al.* "Summarizing data on survival, relapse, and chronic graft-versus-host disease after bone marrow transplantation: Motivation for and description of new methods." *Br. J. Haematol.* **83** (1993): 602–7.

protocol too demanding of their time. Subjects are usually withdrawn by the investigators for safety reasons (a side effect that makes it dangerous for the subject to continue treatment).

Less commonly, investigators may withdraw a subject because they develop a condition that precludes them from participating in one of the arms of the study. For example, in the study of warfarin in atrial fibrillation, the investigators had to withdraw a participant who required valvular replacement during the study. Why? Although valvular replacement does not preclude the development of stroke nor is it a side effect of treatment (or nontreatment), a patient receiving valvular replacement requires anticoagulation with warfarin. Since treatment with warfarin was mandatory, the person could not be continued in a study comparing warfarin to standard treatment.

At first glance, subjects who voluntarily withdraw or are withdrawn by the investigators may seem like losses to follow-up, but there is an important difference. The difference is that withdrawn participants may be willing to let you passively follow them for outcome, even though they do not want to actively participate in your protocol. (This may not be true if they have a side effect and blame you for it!) If the withdrawn subjects will allow you to follow them for outcome, you do not have to censor them prior to the end of the study. Instead you can perform an intention-to-treat analysis.

Intention-to-treat means that participants are counted as members of their originally assigned group, no matter what happens during the study period. For example, in a study with a treatment and a placebo arm, if you perform an intention-to-treat analysis, persons who were assigned to treatment would be part of the treatment group even if they stopped taking the treatment during the study. Intention-to-treat analysis protects against treatments appearing to be more favorable than they are. If subjects with side effects are less likely to benefit from treatment than those without side effects, removing them from the analysis at the time of their side effect will bias your results. It will make your treatment appear more effective than it is. For example, if 100 people are given a new treatment that is effective but causes nausea so severe that only 50 percent of subjects are able to tolerate the treatment long enough to benefit from it, removing 50 study participants will make the treatment look more effective than it is (because a very high proportion of those subjects left in the trial will benefit from the treatment).

The downside of intention-to-treat analysis is that it dilutes the effect of treatment. Keeping to the same example, if you keep 50 subjects who did not take the full treatment in your treatment arm, the treatment arm will be similar to the nontreatment arm. You might ask: Isn't this justified? What good is a treatment if patients cannot tolerate it? But remember there is a difference

DEFINITION

Intention-to-treat means that participants are counted as members of their originally assigned group, no matter what happens during the study period.

between a sample and an individual patient. If I had a terrible disease, I might be interested in trying an efficacious medicine that caused unrelenting vomiting for 50 percent of persons. After all, if I am in the half of persons who doesn't develop vomiting, why should I forgo an efficacious treatment? If the authors only report the results of the intention-to-treat analysis you would not know how efficacious the treatment is for the subgroup of people who can tolerate it. Limiting your analysis to persons who tolerate or comply with treatment is sometimes referred to as an efficacy analysis (how efficacious is the treatment for people who take it?) whereas intention-to-treat analysis is referred to as an effectiveness analysis (how effective is the treatment in the real world?).

TIP

Intention-to-treat is a more conservative approach for estimating the efficacy of treatment than censoring subjects when they withdraw from one of the treatment arms.

If the number of subjects who stop treatment or withdraw from your study is small, it won't matter whether you perform intention-to-treat analysis or censor them at the time they leave the study. Since intention-to-treat is a more conservative approach for estimating the efficacy of treatment than censoring subjects when they withdraw from a treatment arm, most researchers prefer it. In studies where a large number of subjects are withdrawn, you may want to report the analysis both ways.

3.7.D   Varying time of enrollment

Varying times of enrollment (starting times) is an important issue for large prospective studies and for studies of rare diseases. For studies enrolling thousands of participants, logistic constraints preclude everyone from starting the study on the same day. Most large studies are conducted in multiple centers and it is rare for all sites to begin enrollment at the same time. Similarly, with studies of rare diseases it may take several years to identify and enroll enough persons.

In observational studies, varying times of enrollment is the rule, rather than the exception. For example, in the Aerobics Center Longitudinal Study discussed in Section 1.1, the investigators enrolled participants over a 19-year period. Indeed, their study is an open cohort with ongoing accrual of subjects. Subjects are enrolled when they complete the baseline medical examination and are then followed prospectively. Similarly, the investigators of the study of prognosis with melanoma (Section 2.5) included patients who were diagnosed over a nine-year period.

Theoretically, varying start times could be dealt with by following all subjects for a fixed time period (e.g., three years) regardless of when they started the study. In this instance, all subjects who did not drop out, were withdrawn, or experienced the outcome, would have the same length of follow-up. However, this method would decrease the power of the analysis because you would lose the additional follow-up time supplied by the persons who began the study early on. In most studies, the greatest cost (in time and funds) is the initial enrollment and evaluation. The cost of continuing follow-up for the outcome is usually minimal, while the gain, in terms of follow-up time, can be great. Also, waiting until the last enrolled participant completes a preset follow-up period will extend the length of the study often beyond the time that the analytic staff is being supported. Finally, we are all impatient to learn the results of our work. Thus, most investigators will censor results at a common point in calendar time. At this point in time, length of follow-up will differ for the participants. If the longest follow-up is three years, all participants who have follow-up of less than three years and have not experienced an outcome will be censored at the amount of time of follow-up, which in all cases will be less than three years. Those with three years of follow-up and no outcome will be censored at three years.

3.7.E   End of study

> **TIP**
>
> Studies that have a large number of censored observations prior to the end of the study are more problematic than studies that have just a few censored observations.

It may have surprised you that a subject who completes a study (or who in an observational trial has the longest follow-up) without experiencing the outcome is still censored. This is counter-intuitive because in common usage we think of censored subjects as those who do not complete the study. Although all subjects who do not experience the study outcome are ultimately censored, there is an important difference between those censored at the end of a trial and those censored for other reasons. The difference is that for those subjects censored at the end of the study, no assumptions need be made about the future – the study is over. Usually, in the published report, the authors will tell you the date that subjects who completed the study without experiencing an outcome were censored. It is the last date of the study or the last day of observation.

3.8 How can I test the validity of the censoring assumption for my data?

There is no ideal test for assessing the validity of the censoring assumption. It is primarily a judgment call by the investigators, reviewers, and readers of the data. That's why in Section 3.7 I took you through a long discussion of the reasons for censoring and how censored observations may or may not fulfill the assumptions of censoring. Nonetheless, it is possible to make a general assessment about censored observations. First, and foremost, studies that have a large number of censored observations prior to the end of the study are more problematic than studies that have just a few censored observations.

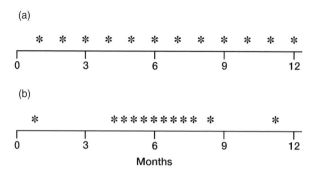

Figure 3.7   Different patterns of censoring. In Figure 3.7(a) censored observations have occurred evenly over the study period, whereas in Figure 3.7(b) censored observations are clumped at 6 months.

Graphical methods, showing when censoring occurred during the trial, can be used to gauge the validity of the censoring assumption. Figures 3.7(a) and 3.7(b) show two very different patterns of censoring. In Figure 3.7(a) it would appear that subjects (shown with asterisks) dropped out evenly through the course of the study. In Figure 3.7(b) it would appear that a clump of subjects dropped out around six months. Whereas the latter suggests some event that occurred at around six months, the former suggests the kind of censoring that you would expect if people dropped out for random reasons such as moving out of town, other obligations, etc.

Graphical displays can also be used to compare censoring in two or more different arms of a study. Figures 3.8(a)–(c) show a treatment and a placebo group. Note how in Figure 3.8(a) the number of persons censored between the treatment and placebo groups is the same and the pattern of censoring between the two groups is also similar. In Figure 3.8(b), the number of censored persons is the same but the pattern between the two groups is different. In Figure 3.8(c), there are many more censored observations in the treatment group. Whereas Figure 3.8(a) is consistent with random censoring, Figures 3.8(b) and 3.8(c) suggest that the causes of censored observations are different for the treatment and placebo group.

A useful method for assessing the validity of the censoring assumption is to compare subjects lost to follow-up to those not lost to follow-up. This can be based on baseline characteristics. So, for example, you can examine whether there are differences by age, race, etc. of persons lost to follow-up compared to persons not lost to follow-up. In particular, you might wish to explore whether subjects at high risk of outcome are differentially lost to follow-up. The censoring assumption can also be tested using time-dependent covariates (Section 9.9.D).

> **TIP**
>
> Censored observations occurring evenly throughout the study are consistent with the censoring assumption, whereas clumps of censored observations suggest nonrandom censoring.

> **TIP**
>
> Similar patterns of censored observations between treatment groups are consistent with the censoring assumption, whereas different patterns suggest nonrandom censoring.

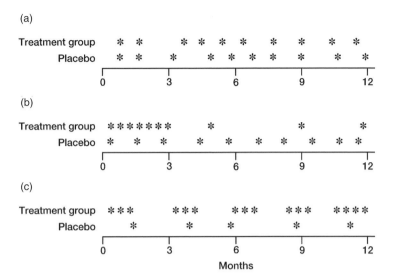

Figure 3.8

Different patterns of censoring between a treatment and a placebo group. In Figure 3.8(a) the patterns of censoring between the two groups are similar. In Figure 3.8(b) there are an equal number of censored observations in the two groups, but the patterns are different. In Figure 3.8(c), there are more censored observations in the treatment group than in the placebo group.

To be certain that censoring owing to alternative outcomes is not affecting your results, report rate of death where possible, in addition to whatever more proximal outcome you are studying. Since there is no alternative outcome to death (no alternative outcome can exclude death), these curves reassure the reader.

For withdrawn cases, it is best to test the censoring assumption by conducting intention-to-treat analyses as described above. Since you may be able to follow withdrawn patients for outcome, you may test whether leaving them in or taking them out makes a difference.

Censoring owing to varying starting times is usually assumed to fulfill the censoring assumptions, since subjects who enroll at the start of a study should be the same as subjects who enroll towards the end. I say "should be" because sometimes investigators become more flexible about the enrollment criteria as studies progress, especially if enrollment is running slowly. Changing the enrollment criteria after a study has begun should be avoided.

But even assuming a group of investigators rigidly used the same enrollment criteria over the course of a long study, one should compare subjects enrolled in the early years of a study to those enrolled in the later years. The reason is that subjects enrolled in later years may be more likely to have received technical advances that were not available in the earlier years of the study. If they were, and these advances could affect development of the outcome of interest, then the assumptions of censoring are not valid.

It is also possible to determine how sensitive your results are to different possibilities of what happened to censored observations. For example, Vittinghoff and colleagues evaluated the impact of multiple risk factors on the occurrence of coronary heart disease among women.[23] Of the sample of 2763 women, 60 were lost to follow-up. The investigators considered two extremes for what could have happened to those women: 1) they had a heart disease event on the day they were censored; 2) their censored date was equal to the longest observed follow-up time. Rerunning their proportional hazards analysis both ways, they found no major changes in the importance/nonimportance of most of the risk factors, with two exceptions: there were changes on the impact of HDL-cholesterol level and smoking on coronary heart disease events.

In conclusion, censoring is a very helpful tool for clinical research. It prevents you from having to delete valuable cases. A randomized controlled trial comparing fluoride to placebo for the prevention of fractures among women with osteoporosis greatly benefited from censoring.[24] Only 135 (67 percent) of the 202 enrolled women were able to complete four years of treatment. If the investigators had deleted these cases they would have lost a third of their sample size. As with any powerful statistical tool, however, censoring should be used carefully. Ask yourself (and tell your reader) the circumstances of persons censored. When you know the outcome of censored cases, perform intention-to-treat analyses.

3.9 What is the proportionality assumption of proportional hazards analysis?

Having reviewed the assumptions underlying censoring, we need to discuss another important assumption of proportional hazards analysis: the proportionality assumption. The assumption is that the hazards for persons with different patterns of covariates are constant over time. In other words, if the relative hazard of heart attack among diabetics is three times higher than among nondiabetics in the first year of the study, the relative hazard of heart attack must also be (about) three times higher among diabetics than nondiabetics in the second year of the study. Note that the hazard for a heart attack

[23] Vittinghoff, E., Shlipak, M. G., Varosy, P. D, *et al.* "Risk factors and secondary prevention in women with heart disease: The heart and estrogen/progestin replacement study." *Ann. Intern. Med.* **138** (2003): 81–9.
[24] Riggs, B. L., Hodgson, S. F., O'Fallon, W. M., *et al.* "Effect of fluoride treatment on the fracture rate in postmenopausal women with osteoporosis." *N. Engl. J. Med.* **322** (1990): 802–9.

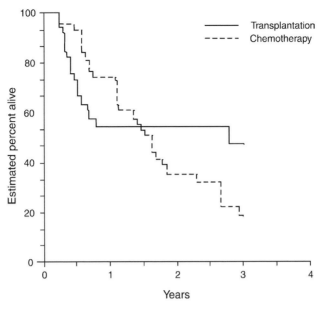

Figure 3.9

Kaplan–Meier curves show the estimated probability of survival for the chemotherapy group (broken line) and the transplantation group (solid line). Reproduced with permission from Appelbaum, F.R., *et al.* "Bone marrow transplantation or chemotherapy after remission induction for adults with acute nonlymphoblastic leukemia." *Ann. Intern. Med.* **101** (1984): 581–8.

can be very different in the first year than in the second year (e.g., much higher in the first year than in the second year), but the difference between the hazards for diabetics and nondiabetics must be constant throughout the study period.

While the proportionality assumption may, at first, sound complicated, it is really very simple. Since proportional hazards analysis, like multiple linear and logistic regression, provides you with a single coefficient for each variable, that coefficient, and its associated relative hazard, must represent the risk throughout the time period. If the risk of outcome associated with a particular variable is higher at one point in time and lower at another, a single coefficient cannot represent that relationship.

For example, in Figure 3.9 we see that the risk of death among patients with acute nonlymphoblastic leukemia was not constant over time in the two arms of the study.[25] Patients who received a bone marrow transplant were more

> **DEFINITION**
>
> The *proportionality assumption* is that the hazards for persons with different patterns of covariates are constant over time.

[25] Appelbaum, F.R., Dahlberg, S., Thomas, E.D., *et al.* "Bone marrow transplantation or chemotherapy after remission induction for adults with acute nonlymphoblastic leukemia." *Ann. Intern. Med.* **101** (1984): 581–8.

likely to die in the first year. But, thereafter, the risk was lower than with conventional chemotherapy.

If you used proportional hazards analysis to analyze the effect of transplantation on death, the relative hazard would probably be one. The higher risk of death associated with transplantation in the first year-and-a-half and the lower risk of death associated with transplantation in the period between a year-and-a-half and three years would average out. Although this average risk of one is arguably the best single estimate of the difference in risk of death with transplantation compared to chemotherapy, you would not want to tell your patients that the risk of death with the two treatments was the same. It would be more informative to tell them that a bone marrow transplant is a toxic treatment and that there are a significant number of deaths caused by it. However, if they survive the treatment, their survival at three years is significantly better than with conventional therapy.

More sophisticated methods of assessing the proportionality assumption, and strategies for analyzing data where the proportionality assumption is not valid, are discussed in Sections 9.9 and 9.10.

3.10 What type of multivariable analysis should I use with counts?

Sometimes a research project will produce count data: for example, the number of hospital admissions or the number of accidents over some period of time. The unit of analysis may be a person (e.g., falls per patient per year), or an institution (e.g., number of admissions per hospital per month), or a population (e.g., number of car accidents per city per day). Usually, the time period for count data will be the same for each unit of analysis, but it is possible to have count data where the time per unit of analysis is different. For example, you can calculate a count variable for number of falls per patient where some patients have been followed for one month to five years. The count for each subject is simply the number of falls (numerator) divided by the number of months of observation for that patient (denominator). In contrast, with incidence rates (Section 3.11) person-time (the denominator) is pooled over the entire population. It is also possible to have counts for community-wide indicators where the numerator is the number of events and the denominator is the number of persons in that community.

As a first pass, you might think that you could analyze this data as an interval outcome. After all, each unit change of a count score has an equal quantifiable value (e.g., the difference between a count of two accidents and four accidents is the same as the difference between three accidents and five accidents). However, unlike an interval variable, with counts there cannot be negative numbers. Also the distribution of counts often does not fit a normal distribution with equal variance. In situations such as these, analyzing the data with a technique such as linear regression is incorrect and the standard errors on which the inferential statistics are based will not be accurate.

What about treating counts as an ordinal variable? This might work if the maximum count is low (e.g., less than four or five) and there are enough observations in each category. But it will not work if there are many different counts and categories with no subjects in them (e.g., if you have 75 subjects and the count can range from 0 to 100, you will have many categories with no subjects; if the person-time of observation varies by subject, you may have no two subjects in the same category). In cases like this you could group the counts (e.g., 0–10 counts equals 1, 11–20 counts equals 2, etc.) but this will result in loss of information.

> Analyze count data with Poisson regression or negative binomial regression.

Instead, with count data whether you are doing a bivariate or multivariable analysis use one of two procedures: Poisson regression or an extension of Poisson regression, negative binomial regression (Table 3.1).[26]

3.10.A Poisson regression

As implied by the name, Poisson regression is based on the Poisson distribution. The Poisson distribution excludes negative numbers, is skewed to the right, and has a variance equal to the mean (Table 3.13). This distribution fits count data from many clinical scenarios because 1) counts cannot have a negative number; 2) counts tend to be skewed to the right since there is no limit to how high a count may go; 3) count data do not generally fit the assumption of equal variance at all values of the independent variable (Section 3.2C). Since negative numbers are not possible with counts, if you have a subgroup with a very low mean you would expect that almost all the values would be equal to zero. This would result in a very small variance. In a different subgroup with a higher mean, you would expect the distribution to be spread across a larger

---

[26] For more on Poisson regression and negative binomial regression see: Hubbard, A. "Modelling counts – The Poisson and negative binomial regression." Available at : http://ehs.sph.berkeley.edu/hubbard/longdata/webfiles/poissonmarch2005.pdf; Kleinbaum, D.G., Kupper, L.L., and Muller, K.E. *Applied Regression Analysis and Other Multivariable Methods* (2nd edn). Boston, MA: PWS-Kent, 1988, pp. 497–512; Gardner, W., Mulvey, E.P., and Shaw, E. "Regression analyses of counts and rates: Poisson, overdispersed Poisson, and negative binomial models." *Psych. Bull.* **118** (1995): 392–404; Simon, S. "Poisson regression model." Available at: http://www.cmh.edu/stats/model/poisson.asp; Grace-Martin, K. "Regression models for count data." StatNews #43, New York, NY: Cornell University, available at: http://www.human.cornell.edu/admin/statcons/statnews/stnews43.htm.

Table 3.13 Underlying assumptions of Poisson and negative binomial regression.

	Poisson	Negative binomial regression
Type of outcome variable	Count or incidence rate	Count or incidence rate
Range of values	Non-negative	Non-negative
What is being modeled	Natural logarithm of outcome	Natural logarithm of outcome
Distribution of outcome	Dependent on the mean	Overdispersed
Variance	Equal to the mean	Variance greater than the mean
Rate of event over time	Constant	Constant

group of values and therefore have a larger variance.[27] Because the Poisson distribution does not assume that the variance is equal in all subgroups but rather that the variance is equal to the mean, the Poisson distribution is often a good fit for count data.

Since Poisson regression models the natural log of the outcome it is sometimes referred to as a log-linear model when it is used to model counts.[28]

A study of the association between income and availability of neighborhood food stores illustrates the value of Poisson regression.[29] The number of stores per persons living in a neighborhood is a count variable (numerator equals number of stores in the neighborhood; denominator equals number of persons living in that neighborhood); this count cannot take on a value less than zero, but could be skewed to the right if some areas have a large number of stores per population.

To assess the association between number of food stores and income the investigators needed to adjust for the density of the area. The reason is that density could confound the relationship between the number of food stores and income; for example, richer people may live in less dense suburbs and lower density encourages placement of more stores (because people don't wish to travel long distances to buy food).

Table 3.14 shows the relationship of income to the count of stores, based on a Poisson regression model adjusted for census tract density (population and tract area size). Note that compared to higher-income tracts, lower-income tracts are less likely to have supermarkets, bakeries, natural food stores, but more likely to have convenience stores, grocery stores, liquor stores, and meat

[27] Gardner, W., Mulvey, E. P., and Shaw, E. "Regression analyses of counts and rates: Poisson, over-dispersed Poisson, and negative binomial models." *Psych. Bull.* **118** (1995): 392–404.
[28] Poisson regression is not referred to as a log-linear model when it is used to analyze rates (Section 3.11).
[29] Moore, L. V. and Roux, A. V. D. "Associations of neighborhood characteristics with the location and type of food stores." *Am. J. Public Health* **96** (2006): 325–31.

Table 3.14 Association between income and presence of food stores.

Type of store	Lowest-income tracts (< $25,000), Ratio (95% CI)	Middle-income tracts ($25,000– $45,000), Ratio (95% CI)	High-income tracts ($45,001– $175,000), Ratio (95% CI)
Supermarkets	0.5 (0.3, 0.8)	0.8 (0.6, 1.0)	1.0 (reference)
Bakeries	0.6 (0.5, 0.8)	0.9 (0.7, 1.1)	1.0 (reference)
Specialty food stores	0.2 (0.1, 0.4)	0.5 (0.3, 0.8)	1.0 (reference)
Natural food stores	0.3 (0.2, 0.5)	0.5 (0.3, 0.8)	1.0 (reference)
Convenience stores	2.4 (1.8, 3.2)	1.6 (1.2, 2.1)	1.0 (reference)
Grocery stores	4.3 (3.6, 5.2)	2.8 (2.3, 3.3)	1.0 (reference)
Liquor stores	1.3 (1.0, 1.6)	0.9 (0.7, 1.2)	1.0 (reference)
Meat and fish markets	2.1 (1.5, 2.8)	1.5 (1.1, 2.1)	1.0 (reference)
Fruit and vegetable markets	0.9 (0.6, 1.4)	0.8 (0.5, 1.2)	1.0 (reference)

Data from Moore, L. V. and Roux, A. V. D. "Associations of neighborhood characteristics with the location and type of food stores." *Am. J. Public Health* **96** (2006): 325–31.

and fish markets. The findings are important because we can't expect people to eat better if there are fewer places to buy fresh fruits and vegetables at affordable prices (e.g., supermarkets).

3.10.B Negative binomial models

> **DEFINITION**
>
> When the variance of a count is much larger than the mean it is called overdispersion.

Sometimes with count data the variance of the count is much larger than the mean. This is referred to as overdispersion. A common situation where this occurs is when there are a large number of zero values (because with many zero values the mean is likely to be very small). In such cases, Poisson regression underestimates the standard errors for the coefficients.

When the variance of the count is greater than the mean, use negative binomial regression (Table 3.13). This technique is a form of Poisson regression that includes a random component with the result that the model may better represent the relationship between the dependent variables and the outcome than a standard Poisson regression when the count is overdispersed.

> **TIP**
>
> When the variance is much larger than the mean, use negative binomial regression.

For example, Leveille and colleagues assessed the association between chronic musculoskeletal pain and falls among older adults.[30] Because the variance is typically greater than the mean with fall data, the authors used negative binomial regression to adjust for potential confounders. The outcome was

[30] Leveille, S. G., Jones, R. N., Kiely, D. K. *et al.* "Chronic musculoskeletal pain and the occurrence of falls in an older population." *JAMA* **302** (2009): 2214–21.

Table 3.15 Association between musculoskeletal pain and falls.

Chronic musculoskeletal pain	
None	1 [Reference]
Single site	1.15 (0.86–1.53)
Polyarticular pain	1.71 (1.33–2.20)

Data from Leveille, S. G., *et al.* "Chronic musculoskeletal pain and the occurrence of falls in an older population." *JAMA* **302** (2009): 2214–21.

the rate of falls, determined by dividing the number of falls of each person by the amount of time each person was followed. As you can see in Table 3.15, older persons with pain, especially with polyarticular pain, had higher rates of falls than elders without pain.

3.11 What type of multivariable analysis should I use with an incidence rate?

TIP

Use Poisson or negative binomial regression with incidence rates.

Incidence rate measures the rate at which a group of people develops a disease or condition(Table 3.1). The numerator is the number of cases of the outcome in a population and the denominator is the observation time for the population (note how this is different than a count variable where the number of events occurring to a person is divided by the observation time of that person – Section 3.10).[31] Often it is of interest to compare incidence rates. For example, we may want to know if the incidence of diabetes is higher in one city than another or is higher among men than women. To perform a simple bivariate comparison of rates we can use the z statistic. However, a z statistic cannot incorporate adjustment for potential confounders. Instead we use Poisson regression and the related procedure negative binomial regression. As is true of counts, incidence rates cannot be negative. Poisson and negative binomial regression are known to fit the incidence of rare diseases particularly well.

You may be wondering if the goal is to compare the incidence of diabetes between two populations why not use proportional hazards analysis. Indeed, this technique would work well if you knew when the observation period began

[31] For more on calculating incidence rates and comparison of incidence rates see: Katz, M. H. *Study Design and Statistical Analysis: A Practical Guide for Clinicians.* Cambridge: Cambridge University Press, 2006, pp. 64–65, 106–7.

for all subjects and when each of them developed the disease. But sometimes when working with population level registries you may not know when the observation period begins for each person, but you may still be able to estimate total observation time.

This point is illustrated by a study examining whether the incidence of stroke is elevated during pregnancy.[32] The investigators used a hospital-based registry in a geographic area to identify strokes in women 15 to 44 years of age. During a three-year period, 31 strokes occurred in women who were pregnant or postpartum (six-week period following pregnancy) and 223 strokes in women who were not pregnant. The person-time at risk during pregnancy was estimated based on the average number of spontaneous and induced abortions, stillbirths, and live births in the population and the average length of each pregnancy state. The person-time not at risk was based on determining the total population of women aged 15 to 44 years of age and subtracting out the estimate of person-time spent pregnant.

The investigators used Poisson regression to adjust for age and race. They found that there was a significantly elevated risk of stroke associated with pregnancy (rate ratio for pregnancy was 2.4; 95% CI = 1.6–3.6), after adjustment for age and race.

Just as occurs with counts (Section 3.10) you may have an incidence rate that is more widely dispersed than the Poisson distribution, for which the mean and the standard deviation are equal. For example, Myers and colleagues studied factors associated with tuberculosis transmission among children 0 to 14 years of age in California.[33] Combining all the census tracts together, the rate of pediatric tuberculosis was 4.1 cases per 100,000 person-years. However, the rates varied widely in different census tracts from 0 to 230 per 100,000 person-years. With widely dispersed rates, the authors appropriately chose negative binomial regression. They found in their multivariable model that Asian race (RR = 1.22; 95% CI = 1.14–1.30), African-American race (RR = 1.19; 95% CI = 1.14–1.23), Hispanic ethnicity (RR = 1.25; 95% CI = 1.12–1.40), foreign birth (RR = 1.26; 95% CI = 1.14–1.40), and low income (RR = 1.62; 95% CI = 1.48–1.78) were associated with higher rates of pediatric tuberculosis. In this multivariable model, crowded housing was associated with a lower rate of pediatric tuberculosis (RR = 0.87; 95% CI = 0.77–0.98). This was the opposite of the finding from the bivariate analysis (RR = 1.59; 95% CI = 1.54–1.64), underscoring the importance of multivariable analysis.

[32] Kittner, S. J., Stern, B. J., Feeser, B. R., *et al.* "Pregnancy and the risk of stroke." *N. Engl. J. Med.* **335** (1996): 768–74.
[33] Myers, W. P., Westenhouse, J. L., Flood, J., Riley, L. W. "An ecological study of tuberculosis transmission in California." *Am. J. Public Health* **96** (2006): 685–90.

A limitation of Poisson and negative binomial regression for comparing incidence rates is that the procedures assume that the probability of an occurrence is constant over time. These techniques are therefore inappropriate for studying occurrences of highly contagious diseases such as chicken pox. (In contrast, proportional hazards analysis (Section 3.6) does not assume that the rate of outcome is constant). Also with incidence rates we are considering only the first occurrence of the event.

3.12 May I change the coding of my outcome variable to use a different type of multivariable analysis?

> Clinicians tend to think dichotomously.

To this point, the focus of this chapter has been on choosing the appropriate type of multivariable analysis based on the nature of your outcome variable. So it may seem that I am throwing you a curved ball in now suggesting the possibility of changing the outcome variable to use a different type of analysis. However, sometimes there are advantages to analyzing your data in a different way, if only to see whether a different method produces similar or different results. The advantages and disadvantages of some commonly performed changes of an outcome variable are listed in Table 3.16 and discussed below.

3.12.A. Dichotomizing an interval variable

As I will discuss more in Chapter 8, the outputs of multiple logistic regression – odds ratios – have an intuitive appeal to clinicians that is not as true of the outputs of multiple linear regression – beta weights. Also, clinicians tend to think dichotomously, even about variables that are inherently interval. For example, clinicians tend to think of a patient as being hypertensive or not, even though blood pressure is an interval variable. For a clinician the difference between a systolic blood pressure of 126 and 136 mm Hg may be unimportant but the difference between a blood pressure of 136 and 146 may be of great importance. In such situations, it may be attractive to dichotomize systolic blood pressure at 140 mmHg and to perform a multiple logistic regression model looking at the factors that significantly increase the risk of hypertension.

A study looking at the impact of parental education on child stunting (linear growth failure owing to poor nutrition and infections) illustrates the practice of dichotomizing interval outcomes to perform logistic regression.[34] As you can see

---

[34] Semba, R. D., de Pee, S., Sun, K., Sari, M., Akhter, N., Bloem, M. W. "Effect of parental formal education on risk of child stunting in Indonesia and Bangladesh: a cross-sectional study." *Lancet* **371** (2008): 322–8.

Table 3.16 Advantages and disadvantages of commonly used changes of an outcome variable so as to perform a different type of multivariable analysis.

Original form of outcome variable	Type of multivariable analysis used for outcome variable	Changed outcome variable	Type of multivariable analysis used for transformed variable	Advantages of change	Disadvantages of change
Interval	Multiple linear regression or ANOVA	Dichotomous	Multiple logistic regression	Results may be more accessible and interpretable for clinicians. Assumptions of normality and equal variance do not need to be met.	Loss of information. Decreased power. Cut-off may be arbitrary.
Time-to-outcome	Proportional hazards analysis	Dichotomous	Multiple logistic regression	Results may be more accessible and interpretable for clinicians. Assumption of proportionality need not be met.	May obscure incremental improvements. Loss of power because multiple logistic regression cannot accommodate censored observations.
Ordinal	Proportional odds regression	Dichotomous	Multiple logistic regression	Results may be more accessible and interpretable for clinicians. Assumption of proportional need not be met.	Loss of information. Decreased power if there is a linear effect.
Ordinal	Proportional odds regression	Nominal	Multinomial logistic regression	Assumption of proportional odds need not be met.	Decreased power if there is a linear effect.
Count	Poisson or negative binomial regression	Time-to-outcome	Proportional hazards analysis	Results may be more accessible and interpretable for clinicians.	Loss of information. Decreased power if there are many people with more than one occurrence.

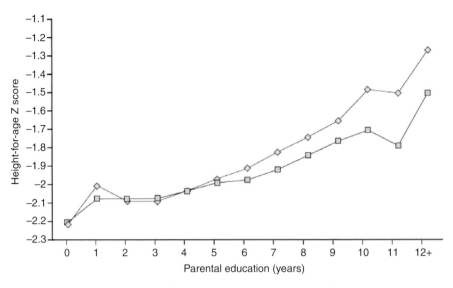

Figure 3.10

Linear relationship between fewer parental years of education and lower height-for-age z score among families living in Bangladesh. Diamonds are for maternal education and squares are for paternal education. Reproduced with permission from Semba, R.D., *et al.* "Effect of parental formal education on risk of child stunting in Indonesia and Bangladesh: a cross-sectional study. " *Lancet* **371** (2008): 322–8.

in Figure 3.10, there is a strong linear relationship between parental education and having a lower height-for-age z score (an interval variable) in Bangladesh. Despite this, rather than use multiple linear regression the authors dichotomized the z score of height-for-age as less than –2 or greater or equal to –2 and used multiple logistic regression. Adjusting for a number of factors, they found that maternal education (years) in a rural setting (odds ratio = 0.950; 95% CI 0.946–954), maternal education (years) in a urban setting (odds ratio = 0.956; 95% CI 0.950–961), and paternal education (odds ratio = 0.970; 95% CI 0.967–974) were all associated with decreased likelihood of stunting.

At times dichotomizing a variable may be a reasonable strategy for dealing with interval outcomes that do not fulfill the assumptions of normality and equal variance, even after they have been transformed (e.g., logarithmic transformation).

Three disadvantages of dichotomizing an interval outcome are 1) loss of information; 2) loss of power; and 3) the cut-off point for dichotomizing the variable may seem to readers (or be!) arbitrary. In the case of the study of stunting, a height-for-age z score is an accepted cut-point. But there is no similarly accepted cut-off for most other variables (e.g., weight, creatinine).

3.12.B. Changing time-to-outcome to a dichotomous outcome (yes/no)

When reading the section on proportional hazards regression you may have wondered if it wouldn't be simpler to analyze the data in terms of the occurrence of an outcome at a particular point in time. In other words, instead of the outcome "time to myocardial infarction" recode it to "myocardial infarction by five years: yes/no." This would have the advantage of enabling you to analyze your data with logistic regression, which is easier to conduct and interpret than proportional hazards analysis. Also, if you used logistic regression analysis, you would not need to worry about meeting the proportionality assumption.

However, there are two major problems with using the simpler dichotomous outcome variable. First, clinical medicine consists more of treatments than of cures. Given this, what matters is not whether or not the disease occurs or recurs, but how soon the disease occurs or recurs.

> **TIP**
>
> Clinical medicine consists more of treatments than of cures.

For example, metastatic colorectal cancer is an extremely deadly disease. Even with chemotherapy the cancer will progress quickly in the majority of patients. Hurwitz and colleagues studied the efficacy of a novel compound, bevacizumab, in patients with metastatic colorectal cancer.[35] Bevacizumab is a monoclonal antibody against vascular endothelial growth factor. The investigators randomized patients to receive either standard chemotherapy with irinotecan, fluorouracil, and leucovorin (IFL) plus placebo, or IFL plus bevacizumab.

As illustrated in Figure 3.11, by 20 months the cancer had progressed in almost all patients in both groups so if you analyzed their data as yes/no survival at 20 months, it will appear that the treatment is ineffective. Yet, the rate of progression between the groups is significantly different. The median progression-free survival is 6.2 months for those who received IFL + placebo, and 10.6 months for those who received IFL + bevacizumab.

One may reasonably ask, especially in these cost-conscious times, how important is it to slow the progression of a disease, if ultimately the same proportion of patients will suffer a recurrence or die? The answer to this question is more philosophical than statistical. In general, time to outcome matters more for serious outcomes than for minor ones. Patients with life-threatening diseases value additional time, whether of days or months, especially if it will allow them to see a child graduate from college or watch a grandchild take her first steps.

---

[35] Hurwitz, H., Fehrenbacher, L., Novotny, W., *et al.* "Bevacizumab plus irinotecan, fluorouracil, and leucovorin for metastatic colorectal cancer." *N. Engl. J. Med.* **350** (2004): 2235–42.

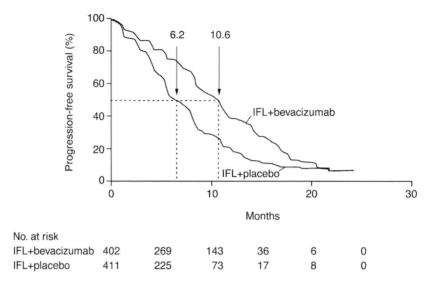

No. at risk
IFL+bevacizumab	402	269	143	36	6	0
IFL+placebo	411	225	73	17	8	0

Figure 3.11   Kaplan–Meier estimates of progression-free survival. Although the cancer progresses in almost all patients in both groups by 20 months, the patients who received bevacizumab progressed more slowly. Figure is from Hurwitz, H., Fehrenbacher, L., Novotny, W., *et al.* "Bevacizumab plus irinotecan, fluorouracil, and leucovorin for metastatic colorectal cancer." *N. Engl. J. Med.* **350** (2004): 2235–42. Copyright 2004, Massachusetts Medical Society. All rights reserved.

TIP

Time to outcome matters more for serious outcomes than for minor ones.

At the other extreme, for minor outcomes, increased time may not be clinically meaningful. For example, studies have shown that children with chicken pox treated with acyclovir have one day less fever, and experience a decrease in the number of chicken pox lesions one day sooner than those given placebo.[36] If the investigators had used symptoms at seven days as the outcome of their study they would have found no effect for acyclovir because, treated or untreated, immunocompetent children with chicken pox are almost invariably well at seven days. Is it worth the expense of acyclovir for one day less of symptoms? Is it worth the trouble (those of you who have attempted to give a toddler a medicine four times a day know what I mean)? Clearly, this is not a statistical question. In practice, most pediatricians do not prescribe acyclovir for immunocompetent children.

At times, small improvements in the time to outcome may spur scientific progress, even if there is minimal benefit to individual patients. Most medical advances are incremental. Proving that a particular strategy

---

[36] Balfour, H. H., Kelly, J. M., Suarez, C. S., *et al.* "Acyclovir treatment of varicella in otherwise healthy children." *J. Pediatr.* **116** (1990): 633–99.

increases survival, if only marginally, may provide a valuable lead to a better treatment.

A second reason for not using logistic regression analysis in place of proportional hazards analysis is that the former procedure cannot accommodate censored observations. Subjects who are withdrawn from the trial, lost to follow-up, etc. will need to be excluded from a logistic regression analysis. This may result in a substantial loss of power, if a large number of subjects have to be excluded. Excluding subjects may also introduce bias into the study if the subjects who are excluded from the final analysis are different from those who remain in the study.

> Logistic regression and proportional hazards analysis are likely to produce similar answers when there are relatively few outcomes, follow-up is relatively short, and few subjects are lost.

Overall, studies using both logistic regression and proportional hazards analysis have found that if you have relatively few outcomes, length of follow-up is relatively short, and few subjects are lost to follow-up, then logistic regression will provide similar results as proportional hazards analysis.[37] For example, Kravitz and colleagues assessed the impact of coronary revascularization on mortality.[38] Of 671 patients, 70 (10.4%) were known to have died, the median follow-up was 797 days, and mortality data were available for all subjects. Multiple logistic regression, adjusted for a number of potential confounders, showed that the odds of death at one year were significantly lower among patients who received coronary revascularization (OR = 0.49; 95% CI = 0.30–0.84) compared to those who did not receive it. A proportional hazards analysis, which also adjusted for confounders, found that revascularization significantly reduced the risk of death (relative hazard [RH] = 0.59; 95% CI = 0.36–0.97).

3.12.C Dichotomizing ordinal variables or treating them as nominal variables

Because ordinal outcomes are infrequently used with multivariable analysis, it is common to dichotomize them and use logistic regression. For example, New York Heart Association classification is often grouped as level I and II (mild shortness of breath) or level III and IV (severe shortness of breath). The advantage is that readers better understand logistic regression than proportional odds regression. Also, with logistic regression the proportional odds assumption need not be met. The disadvantage, as is true of dichotomizing an interval variable, is loss of information and power and the arbitrary nature of any cut-off.

---

[37] Green, M. S. and Symons, M. J. "A comparison of the logistic risk function and the proportional hazards model in prospective epidemiologic studies." *J. Chron. Dis.* **36** (1983): 715–24.

[38] Kravitz, R. L., Laouri, M., Kahan, J. P., *et al.* "Validity of criteria used for detecting under- use of coronary revascularization." *JAMA* **274** (1995): 632–8.

Another option with ordinal variables is to treat them as nominal variables (essentially ignoring the inherent ordering in them) and to use multinomial logistic regression to analyze them. The advantage of this approach is that the proportional odds assumption need not be met. For example, Galanis and colleagues assessed the impact of alcohol intake on cognitive function.[39] Cognitive function was measured using an established scale with a range of 0 to 100. The distribution of scores did not fit a normal distribution – they were skewed with most scores on the high end. The investigators handled this issue in two different ways. They used a (cubic) mathematical transformation (Section 4.3.A) that resulted in an approximately normal distribution and maintained the interval nature of the variable. They also transformed the variable into an ordinal scale by trichotomizing it (dividing it into terciles – or 3 groups): good cognition (score > 82), intermediate cognition (score 74 –81), and poor cognition (score < 74).

Although the trichotomized version of their cognitive measure was an ordinal scale, in their multivariable analysis the investigators treated it as a nominal variable and used multinomial regression analysis. The results are shown in Table 3.17. The good cognition group is the reference. There are two sets of risk ratios for each category change in alcohol consumption. The risk ratios on the 2nd row show you the change in risk between the intermediate cognition function group and the good cognition function group as you increase alcohol consumption. The risk ratios on the fifth row show you the change in risk between the poor cognitive function group and the good group as you increase alcohol consumption.

Had the authors used proportional odds regression there would have been only one set of risk ratios representing the average of the change in cognitive function as alcohol consumption increased. Because they used multinomial regression their data need not fulfill the proportional odds assumption. Of course, anytime you treat an ordinal variable as nominal you will decrease the power of your analysis to detect a statistically significant linear relationship.

3.12.D.   Converting a count to time to outcome or to a dichotomous outcome

Some count variables are actually dichotomous variables that can occur more than once over time. For example, if you look back at the study of the impact of musculoskeletal pain on falls (Section 3.10), you will see that the count variable

---

[39] Galanis, D. J., Joseph, C., Masaki, K. H., Petrovitch, H., Ross, G. W., White, L. "A longitudinal study of drinking and cognitive performance in elderly Japanese American men: The Honolulu – Asia Aging Study." *Am. J. Public Health* **90** (2000): 1254–9.

Table 3.17 Association of alcohol intake with cognitive function score, trichotomized as poor, intermediate, and good score.

	Alcohol intake (oz/mo)					
	None	1–2	3–15	16–30	31–60	>60
Intermediate vs. good cognitive function						
Number interm./good scores	180/634	107/546	155/676	65/241	46/208	39/123
Risk ratio	1.00	0.78	0.89	0.89	0.68	1.02
95% confidence interval		0.59, 1.03	0.69, 1.15	0.64, 1.25	0.46, 1.00	0.67, 1.55
Poor vs. good cognitive function						
Number poor/good scores	182/634	98/546	95/676	56/241	57/208	48/123
Risk ratio	1.00	0.74	0.60	0.72	0.78	1.29
95% confidence interval		0.54, 1.01	0.44, 0.82	0.49, 1.06	0.52, 1.17	0.83, 2.01

Data from Galanis, D. J., *et al.* "A longitudinal study of drinking and cognitive performance in elderly Japanese American men: The Honolulu–Asia Aging Study." *Am. J. Pub. Health* **90** (2000): 1254–9.

"falls" consists of a dichotomous variable (fall: yes/no) divided by the observation time for each person. If we were to look at only the first occurrence of the outcome, we could use proportional hazards regression to determine time to outcome, and the relative hazards of falls for persons with or without musculoskeletal pain. The advantage is that this procedure is more familiar to readers than Poisson or negative binomial regression. The disadvantage is that unless the majority of subjects have no falls or only one fall, we would lose a great deal of information. We could also simplify this outcome even further to a fall (yes/no) for each subject within a certain period of time and use multiple (binary) logistic regression. In this case, we would not only lose information owing to repeated falls, but would also be unable to accommodate subjects who were lost to follow-up or censored for some other reason.

3.12.E General advice for changing the coding of outcome variables

> Demonstrating similar results with different analytic methods strengthens your findings.

In general it is best to analyze data fully, to not simplify outcomes in order to use simpler analytic techniques. On the other hand, changing the nature of your outcome variable is often the best alternative when assumptions are not met. Also, demonstrating similar results with different analytic methods strengthens your findings.

Independent variables in multivariable analysis

4.1 How do I incorporate my independent variables into a multivariable analysis?

Having determined, based on your outcome variable, the type of multivariable analysis you will be doing (Chapter 3), it is now time to consider how you will enter your independent variables into your multivariable model. While dichotomous variables can be entered into all multivariable analyses without special coding or transformation, there are special considerations for the treatment of nominal, interval, and ordinal independent variables. These are considered in Sections 4.2–4.4.

4.2 How do I incorporate nominal independent variables into a multivariable analysis?

Nominal independent variables, such as race or type of cancer, cannot be entered into a multivariable analysis, unless they are transformed. The reason is that the numeric codings for the variables have no meaning. You may have coded your variable 1 = Caucasian, 2 = African-American, but the numbers don't reflect a meaningful order. Therefore, any multivariable estimate of the change of going from one category to another is meaningless.

To incorporate a nominal independent variable into a multivariable model you must transform it into multiple dichotomous variables. This process is usually called "dummying" by epidemiologists and biostatisticians. However, the terms "dummying" and "dummy variables" are slang. In manuscripts, you should refer to this process as creating multiple categorical variables (if you refer to it as dummying, you may, as I did, receive complaints from the reviewers of your article).

> **TIP**
>
> To incorporate nominal variables into a multivariable model transform it into multiple dichotomous variables.

Ethnicity is probably the most common nominal variable in clinical research. (You will remember I used ethnicity as an example for a nominal dependent variable in Section 3.5). When ethnicity is used as an independent variable in multivariable analysis it should be represented as several

Table 4.1 Creation of multiple dichotomous variables to represent a nominal independent variable.

	African-American	Latino/Hispanic	Asian/Pacific Islander	Native American	Other nonwhite
African-American	1	0	0	0	0
Latino/Hispanic	0	1	0	0	0
Asian/Pacific Islander	0	0	1	0	0
Native American	0	0	0	1	0
Other nonwhite	0	0	0	0	1
White/Caucasian	0	0	0	0	0

dichotomous variables. For example, ethnicity can be represented as five dichotomous variables:

African-American (yes/no)
Latino/Hispanic (yes/no)
Asian/Pacific Islander (yes/no)
Native American (yes/no)
Other nonwhite (yes/no)

What happened to persons who are white/Caucasian? When you represent a nominal variable as several dichotomous variables in multivariable analysis you need one variable less than the number of categories of your variable. Why? To answer this question, think about it from the computer's point of view. If you create five dichotomous variables, all of which are either 1 (yes) or 0 (no), the computer will see six patterns as shown in Table 4.1.

We don't create a variable white/Caucasian because it is represented by the other five variables (zero on all five variables). In multivariable analysis, this is called a reference group.

Ethnicity is an interesting example of a nominal variable because how you choose to code it will depend on your study population. For example, in a small clinical study performed in the southeast of the United States, there may be very few Native Americans or Asian/Pacific Islanders. If a group represents less than 5 percent of the total sample, creating a variable for that group may not carry much statistically important information. In this case you might only create variables for the larger ethnic groups and then have a group that is "other." For example, your variables would be African-American (yes/no), Latino/Hispanic (yes/no), and other nonwhite ethnicity (yes/no), with white as the reference group.

Although decreasing the number of groups may prevent having dichotomous variables that convey little information, grouping people of different

TIP

The best way to group a nominal variable will depend on the research question, the distribution of the nominal variable, and the bivariate relationship between the nominal variable and the outcome.

ethnicities in one group may not adequately represent the data. Even if you retain the category "Asian/Pacific Islander" remember that this category contains more than a dozen disparate cultures, each with their own language, traditions, and genetic composition, all of which could affect the development of disease. As with all really hard questions in multivariable analysis, the question of how to code ethnicity is not a statistical question. The best way to group a nominal independent variable such as ethnicity will depend on the research question, the distribution of the nominal variable (how many people are in each group), and the relationship between the different categories of the nominal variable and the outcome.

4.3 How do I incorporate interval-independent variables into a multivariable model?

As you will remember, each unit of an interval variable is equal. Therefore, a multivariable model will assume that a unit change anywhere on the scale of the interval variable will have an equal effect on the modeled outcome. For example, the change due to a 10 kg weight gain on the dependent variable is the same whether it is from 50 kg to 60 kg or 90 kg to 100 kg. However, the change in the outcome of a given change of an interval variable (say 10 kg) varies with the different multivariable models because of differences in what is being modeled. For example, with a linear regression model, an equal size change of an interval-independent variable will have an equal size change to the mean value of the outcome; with a logistic regression, an equal size change of an interval-independent variable will have an equal size change to the logit of the outcome; with a proportional hazards analysis an equal size change of an independent variable will have an equal size change to the logarithm of the relative hazard.

The linearity
assumption is that an
equal change of an
interval-independent
variable will have
an equal effect on
outcome.

The assumption that an equal change of an interval-independent variable will have an equal effect on outcome is referred to as the linearity assumption, and is easiest to appreciate in the case of linear regression. If the linearity assumption is true, then a scatter plot of the two variables should show a line. For example, look back at Figure 3.1. It is a scatter plot of the relationship of two interval variables. A line fits the data because equal increases in the values of B_{12} anywhere along the scale are associated with equal increases in titers after vaccine.

TIP

The linearity assumption for linear regression is tested by performing a scatter plot of your raw independent variable versus your outcome variable.

However, sometimes a scatter plot will not show a linear relationship. For example, Figure 4.1(a) is an illustration of a logarithmic relationship between an independent variable and an outcome. At the low end of the scale changes in the independent variable are associated with very large changes in the

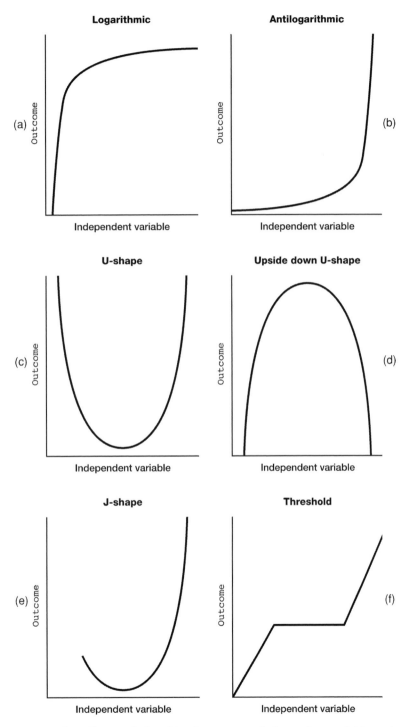

Figure 4.1   Variety of nonlinear relationships between an independent variable and an outcome.

outcome; at the high end of the scale, changes in the independent variable have very little effect on the outcome.

A variety of nonlinear relationships are possible. Some common ones, in addition to logarithmic, are: antilogarithmic, curvilinear (**U**-shape, upside down **U**–shape, **J**-shape), and threshold.

A limitation of the use of a bivariate scatter plot to determine linearity is that it is possible for a relationship between an interval-independent variable and an interval outcome to be linear in a bivariate analysis but not in a multiple linear regression analysis owing to confounding. Methods of testing for linear relationships in multiple linear regression models are described in Section 9.4.

To assess whether an interval variable fits the linear assumption of logistic regression (or the closely related techniques of proportional odds regression and multinomial regression), proportional hazards analysis, and Poisson regression (or the closely related technique of negative binomial regression), you cannot assess the linear assumption by making a simple scatter plot. This is because the linear relationship does not exist on a simple arithmetic scale. Instead, categorize the interval variable into multiple dichotomous variables (Section 4.2) of equal units on the variable's scale. So, for example, if the variable you are testing is age, and the ages of your subjects range from 20 to 79, have age 20–29 be your reference group. Then create variables 30–39 (yes/no), 40–49 (yes/no), 50–59 (yes/no), 60–69 (yes/no), and 70–79 (yes/no). If you would have too few subjects being yes in these decade categories, you can group them into 20-year periods.

> **TIP**
> To assess whether an interval variable fits the linear assumption of logistic regression, proportional hazards analysis, or Poisson regression: (1) Categorize the variable into multiple dichotomous variables of equal units; (2) enter these dichotomous variables in the analysis; and (3) graph each variable's coefficient against the midpoint of the variable.

Perform the logistic or proportional hazards or Poisson analysis with these several dichotomous variables. Each variable will have an estimated coefficient. The coefficient for the reference group is, by definition, 0. Graph the coefficient against the midpoint of each dichotomous variable (e.g., 35 years for the variable that represents the 30–39 group). The graph will show you the relationship between your independent and outcome variable. If you have a linear effect, the coefficients will steadily increase (or decrease) as you go from one age group to another, and you will get a straight line (as shown in Figure 4.2). Alternatively, your graph may appear like one of the nonlinear relationships in Figure 4.1.

Even without graphing, if you have a linear effect, you should be able to see it because the numeric difference between the coefficients of each successive group should be about equal (e.g., the numeric difference between the coefficient of the 30–39 group and the coefficient of the 20–29 group will be equal to the difference between the coefficient of the 40–49 variable and the 30–39 variable). Remember, of course, they are not going to be exactly equal (just as the points do not fall exactly on a straight line). The important issue is whether the data can be reasonably expressed as a linear relationship.

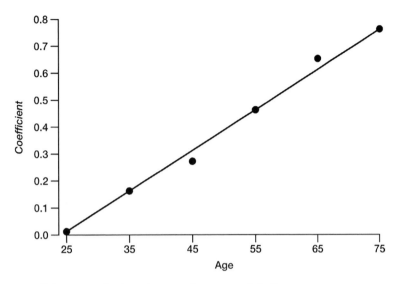

Figure 4.2   Coefficients graphed against age form a straight line.

This technique can be used to determine whether a linear relationship exists between an independent variable and an outcome variable after adjustment for potential confounders. Besides being useful for testing a linear association, this technique is also useful for demonstrating a linear dose–response curve between an independent variable and outcome.[1] Plots of residuals are also helpful in determining whether a variable fulfills the linearity assumption; they are described in Section 9.4.

There is another bivariate method of assessing whether an interval-independent variable has a linear association with the outcome that can be done prior to logistic regression. It requires grouping your interval-independent variable data into categories that preserve the interval nature of the variable (e.g., 1 = ages 20–29, 2 = ages 30–39, 3 = ages 40–49, etc.) and are large enough to provide a reasonable number of outcomes in each category. You can then perform a simple cross-tabulation of your independent variable and outcome. The cross-tabulation table should show a steadily increasing (or decreasing) proportion of outcomes as you increase (or decrease) along the levels of your interval-independent variable. The chi-squared for trend test should be significant. A bar graph can demonstrate the same trend visually.

---

[1] If you are unfamiliar with multiple logistic regression and proportional hazards analysis, this section will make more sense to you after you have read Section 8.3 on interpretation of coefficients. For a more detailed explanation of this technique see: Hosmer, D. W. and Lemeshow, S. *Applied Logistic Regression*. 2nd edn. New York, NY: Wiley, 2000, pp. 110–11.

Table 4.2 Methods for incorporating interval-independent variables into a multivariable model when they do not have a linear relationship with outcome.

Method	Advantages	Disadvantages
Mathematical transformation	Simple to perform	May be difficult to interpret clinically. There may not be a mathematical transformation that captures the relationship between the interval-independent variable and the outcome
Splines	Can model complex relationships between the interval-independent variable and the outcome	Does not result in a single measure of the association of the independent variable with the outcome. Difficult for many nonstatisticians to understand
Multiple dichotomous variables	Easy to interpret	Choice of cut-offs may be arbitrary. Loss of the interval nature of the variable

If your interval-independent variable does not have a linear relationship with your outcome, don't be discouraged. You have learned something important about the relationship of your variables. Three options for incorporating nonlinear relationships are shown in Table 4.2 and discussed below.

4.3.A Mathematical transformations

The simplest method of incorporating an interval-independent variable that does not have a linear relationship with outcome is to transform it so that it does fulfill the linearity assumption. For example, if changes in value at the high end of your independent variable have less impact on your outcome variable than changes at the lower end (as indicated by a steadily decreasing slope), with the high end of the independent variable asymptotically approaching a horizontal level as in Figure 4.1(a), a logarithmic transformation of the independent variable (the logarithm of the variable) may linearize the trend. The natural logarithm is used more often than the logarithm to the base 10, although both may linearize the effect. Remember that with either logarithmic transformation, values for the variable must be positive (i.e., you cannot take the logarithm of zero or negative numbers). If your scale has a true zero you can still use a logarithmic transformation by adding one to all values.

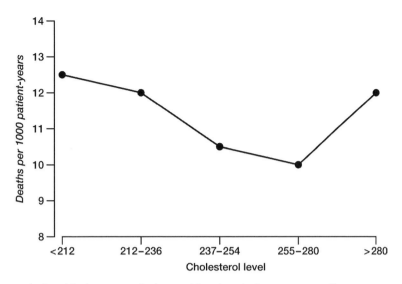

Figure 4.3   Relationship between cholesterol level and all-cause mortality among 1102 women. Adapted with permission from: Isles, C.G., *et al.* "Plasma cholesterol, coronary heart disease, and cancer in the Renfrew and Paisley survey." *Br. Med. J.* **298** (1989): 920–4. Copyright BMJ Publishing Group.

If changes in value at the high end of your independent variable have a greater impact on your outcome variable than changes at the lower end (as indicated by a steadily increasing slope as in Figure 4.1(b)), an antilogarithm transformation (i.e., e^x or 10^x) of the independent variable may linearize the trend. Logarithmic or antilogarithmic transformations can be made of the independent or dependent variable.[2]

At times you may find that there is a **U**-shaped relationship between your interval-independent variable and your outcome. For example, Figure 4.3 shows a **U**-shaped relationship between cholesterol level and all-cause mortality in a sample of 1102 women.[3] Mortality is highest for women with the lowest and the highest values of cholesterol. When the investigators treated cholesterol as an interval variable, there was no significant relationship between cholesterol level and mortality, because the two trends statistically cancel each other out. Treating cholesterol as an interval variable misses the vital information contained in the curvilinear relationship: High cholesterol levels are associated with increased mortality from coronary artery disease, whereas low

[2] Other mathematical transformations are possible: See: Armitage,P. and Berry,G. *Statistical Methods in Medical Research* (2nd edn). Oxford: Blackwell Scientific Publications, 1987, pp. 358–68.

[3] Isles, C.G., Hole, D.J., Gillis, C.R., Hawthorne, V.M., Lever, A.F. "Plasma cholesterol, coronary heart disease, and cancer in the Renfrew and Paisley survey." *Br. Med. J.* **298** (1989): 920–4.

levels of cholesterol are associated with increased mortality from cancer and other causes.

TIP

When you note a **U**-shaped relationship consider creating a quadratic form of the variable.

When you note a **U**-shaped relationship consider creating a quadratic form of the variable. To create the quadratic form of a variable first subtract out the mean of the untransformed variable (X) and then square the result: (value of X – mean of X for sample). Now enter both the quadratic form of the variable, and the untransformed variable into the model. The untransformed variable must be in the model because the quadratic term is comparing extremes to the mean of the untransformed variable. Large differences from the mean in either direction cause the term to be statistically significant. If the relationship is **U**-shaped both terms will be statistically significant in your model.

A quadratic form of a variable will also work with a **J**-shaped relationship. As you can tell from Figure 4.1(e), a **J**-shaped curve is just like a **U**-shaped curve with a few missing data points.

A limitation of the use of mathematical transformations is that they can be difficult to interpret. For example, what would it mean to a practicing clinician to know that the logarithm of the cholesterol level was associated with increased mortality? Quadratic terms can be particularly difficult to interpret because a unit change in the interval-independent factor affects the outcome through two variables – each with a different relationship with the outcome. However, the greatest weakness of mathematical transformations is that for many associations there is no simple mathematical transformation that will fulfill the linearity assumption. This brings us to splines.

4.3.B Splines

DEFINITION

Splines are polynomials linked together; they are used to model complex relationships between interval-independent variables and outcomes.

Splines enable us to model complex relationships between interval-independent variables and outcomes.[4] The term spline originates from the flexible strip of metal used by draftsmen to draw curves. In the statistical sense, splines are polynomials (an algebraic function of two or more summed terms) that are connected to one another. The points at which they are connected are called knots. Because each piece of the curve is represented by a different polynomial, splines can be used to model a variety of complex relationships.

The simplest type of spline is a linear spline function. Although each piece of the function is linear, because you have multiple pieces, you can model non-linear relationships between interval-independent variables and outcomes. For example, Figure 4.3 could be modeled as a linear spline function consisting of

---

[4] For a very lucid explanation of splines see: Harrell, F. E. *Regression Modeling Strategies: With Applications to Linear Models, Logistic Regression, and Survival Analysis.* New York: Springer-Verlag, 2001, pp. 18–24.

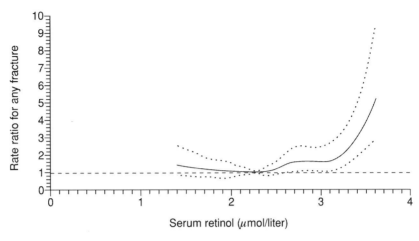

Figure 4.4

Smoothed plots of rate ratios (solid line) and 95% confidence intervals (dotted lines) for having a fracture according to the serum retinol level. Plot based on use of restricted cubic splines and Cox regression analysis. Figure is from Michaelsson, K., Lithell, H., Vessby, B., *et al.* "Serum retinol levels and the risk of fracture." *N. Engl. J. Med.* **348** (2003): 287–94. Copyright 2003 Massachusetts Medical Society. All rights reserved.

four linear segments. (If Figure 4.3 were a spline function it would have three knots at the cholesterol levels 212–236, 237–254, and 255–280; these are the points where the segments touch. The number of knots will always be one less than the number of segments.)

When modeling the relationship between a risk factor and an outcome you may find that not all the pieces are linear. Instead, you may have rounded curves. In this case you should use a cubic spline function. Because cubic spline functions are higher-order polynomials they better approximate curves.

A weakness of cubic spline functions is that they may not perform well at the tails (before the first knot and after the last knot). To overcome this problem use a restricted cubic spline function (also referred to as a natural cubic spline), which constrains the function to be linear beyond the boundary knots. The restricted cubic spline function also requires fewer parameters to be estimated than the cubic spline function.

Michaelsson and colleagues used a restricted cubic spline function and proportional hazards analysis to assess the relationship between serum retinol levels and the risk of bone fracture.[5] As you can see in Figure 4.4 the relationship

TIP

For rounded curves use a restricted cubic spline function.

[5] Michaelsson, K., Lithell, H., Vessby, B., *et al.* "Serum retinol levels and the risk of fracture." *N. Engl. J. Med.* **348** (2003): 287–94.

between serum retinol level and fracture rate is not linear. In particular, the rate of fractures increases sharply at higher levels of retinol. As was done in this figure, splines can be smoothed.

Although statistically splines are a very satisfying solution, they are only slowly catching on in the medical literature. The major reason is that splines do not result in a single measure (e.g., odds ratio, relative risk) of the association of a risk factor with an outcome (as you would get if you treated the variable as if the association were linear). Also, they are difficult for nonstatisticians to understand.

4.3.C Multiple dichotomous variables

The third method for incorporating nonlinear relationships between an interval risk factor and an outcome in a multivariable model is to create multiple dichotomous variables from the interval variable. This is the same procedure as you would use for incorporating a nominal variable into your analysis (Section 4.2) or for testing whether an interval-independent variable has a linear relationship with the outcome (Section 9.4). Multiple dichotomous variables allow each category to be its own independent variable and have its own relationship to the outcome.

For example, in the study of serum retinol levels and fracture risks described above, the authors demonstrated their results using multiple dichotomous variables in addition to the analysis with a restricted cubic spline function. The results are shown in Table 4.3.

The risk of fracture is 1.64 times higher among persons in the highest quintile level compared with those in the middle quintile. You can see that presenting relative risks associated with the different quintiles of the serum retinol level tells the same story as the cubic spline function, but much less elegantly.

One of the major challenges with using multiple dichotomous variables is determining the cut-offs. In general, it is best to use cut-offs that reflect a natural, clinically relevant standard. For example, with systolic blood pressure, sensible cut-offs would be < 90 mm, 90–140 mm, >140 mm.

A disadvantage of choosing natural cut-offs, is that the cut-offs may divide the sample into groups with unequal sample sizes. For example, if you divide your sample into decades of age, you may only have 2 percent of your sample as "yes" on the variable 80–89 years. If the number of persons who are yes on this variable is too small, the variable will not be meaningful in the analysis. In comparison, if you choose cut-offs that provide equal sample sizes then the distributions of the multiple dichotomous variables will be equal. For example,

> **TIP**
>
> Choose cut-off points by using natural cut-offs if they are available.

Table 4.3 Rate ratio for any fracture according to the base-line serum retinol level.

Retinol quintile	Multivariate RR* (95% CI)
1 (<1.95 µmol/liter)	0.93 (0.62–1.41)
2 (1.95–2.16 µmol/liter)	0.78 (0.50–1.23)
3 (2.17–2.36 µmol/liter)	1.00 (reference)
4 (2.37–2.64 µmol/liter)	0.91 (0.60–1.38)
5 (>2.64 µmol/liter)	1.64 (1.12–2.41)

* The analysis was adjusted for age, weight, height, and serum beta carotene, calcium, and albumin values (all continuous variables); smoking status (never smoked, former smoker, or current smoker); marital status (married or living with a partner vs. single); socioeconomic class (low, middle, or high); and physical activity at work, leisure physical activity, and alcohol consumption (all in three categories).
Data from: Michaelsson, K., *et al.* "Serum retinol levels and the risk of fracture." *N. Engl. J. Med.* **348** (2003): 287–94.

let's assume you divide the sample into terciles of age and make the youngest people the reference group. One dichotomous variable will have a "yes" value for a third of the sample (the middle-aged people) and a "no" value for two thirds of the sample (the youngest and oldest persons); the other dichotomous variable will also have a "yes" value for a third of the sample (the oldest persons) and a "no" value for two-thirds of the sample (the youngest and the middle-aged persons).

One method for assuring equal-sized groups is to choose cut-offs based on an equal distribution of subjects, such as terciles, quartiles, quintiles of values of the independent variable, as was done in the study of serum retinol levels and fractures. While this guarantees groups of equal sizes, dropping the natural units of the independent variable may make your results sound less compelling. Which of the following sounds more compelling? Persons in the highest tercile of age are three times more likely to die than persons in the lowest tercile of age, or persons aged 70–89 years are three times more likely to die than persons aged 30–49 years. The latter sounds more compelling. Don't you think?

Regardless of the method of choosing cut-offs a downside of using multiple dichotomous variables to represent an interval variable is that they increase the number of variables in your model. This can be a problem if you do not have a large enough sample size (Section 6.5).

4.4 Assuming that my interval-independent variable fits a linear assumption, is there any reason to group it into interval categories or create multiple dichotomous variables?

Even when an interval-independent variable, such as age, blood pressure, or cholesterol, fits the linear assumption it is often not left in its original interval form. There are several reasons for this.

For one thing, if you have a small sample size (e.g., 100 persons) it may be difficult to evaluate whether an interval variable (e.g., age) fits the linear assumption unless you group it into categories. Left ungrouped your model will assume that the difference in the likelihood of outcome between a subject age 55 and a subject age 57 is the same as that between a subject age 61 and a subject age 63. Yet you may have no one or just one or two persons in your entire sample with these ages. Also, your audience is likely to be more interested in the impact of ten years on outcome, than the impact of a single year (which is likely to be very small for most diseases).

When grouping an interval variable maintain the interval nature of the scale (e.g., group age by decades). This will allow you to retain the advantages of an interval scale (because the difference between being 20–29, 30–39, and 40–49, etc. is the same – 10 years). Yet, you will be better able to assess whether the variable fits the assumptions of the statistical model and you will be able to report a more meaningful result.

> **TIP**
>
> When grouping interval variables maintain the interval nature of the scale.

Sometimes researchers create multiple dichotomous variables even though the variable approximates a linear relationship. The reason is that creation of multiple dichotomous variables is a more conservative strategy. Since a linear relationship is not assumed, you do not have to prove to your readers (or your reviewers!) that the linear assumption is fulfilled. However, this strategy results in an increase in the number of variables in your model; this may be a problem if your sample size is small (Section 6.5). Also a statistically significant linear trend between an interval risk factor and an outcome may no longer appear to be statistically significant when the interval variable is represented as multiple dichotomous variables because none of the variables themselves is significantly different from the reference group.

4.5 How do I incorporate ordinal independent variables into a multivariable model?

Ordinal variables pose a challenge similar to nominal variables when used as independent variables in a multivariable model. Because there is not an equal distance between each level of an ordinal variable, having a single estimate of the impact of moving from one level of the variable to another on a dependent variable may not be accurate, and therefore you should create multiple dichotomous variables. On the other hand, there may be variables that are technically ordinal in nature but can be treated as if they are interval because they operate as if they are ordinal. In other words, a single estimate of an equal change anywhere along the scale is valid. This is often the case for interval measures based on psychological and sociological scales that are derived from multiple questions (Section 6.5.C.3).

Relationship of independent variables to one another

5.1 Does it matter if my independent variables are related to each other?

As discussed in Section 1.1, the strength of multivariable analysis is its ability to determine how multiple independent variables, which are related to one another, are related to an outcome. We would not need multivariable analysis to determine the independent effect of exercise on mortality if it weren't for the fact that exercise, smoking, age, hypertension, and cholesterol level were all related to each other and the outcome of interest. Multivariable analysis helps us to separate the effects of these different variables on outcomes such as mortality.

However, if two variables are so closely correlated that if you know the value for one variable you know the value of the other, multivariable analysis cannot separately assess the impact of these two variables on the outcome. This problem is called multicollinearity.[1] I can best illustrate it with an extreme example.

Let's say you were studying factors that affected length of hospital stay among patients with pneumonia. At your hospital, to accommodate the different preferences of the staff, the nurses record patients' temperature in both Fahrenheit and Celsius. When you do your medical abstraction, you record both Fahrenheit and Celsius temperatures. If you entered both variables in a model assessing length of stay, your model would be incorrect, and you would get an error message or unpredictable answers. This is because temperature in Celsius and temperature in Fahrenheit is the same variable even though the numbers are different. There is a simple mathematical conversion from one to the other: Celsius = (Fahrenheit − 32) × 0.56.

---

[1] Some authors distinguish between collinearity – two variables that are highly related to one another – and multicollinearity – more than two variables that are highly related to one another. More commonly, both situations are lumped as multicollinearity, and this is the term I use throughout the book.

Your model cannot possibly assess the independent contribution of temperature in Fahrenheit and in Celsius because they are really the same variable. However, unless you make a mistake and include two variables that really are the same variable (such as temperature in Fahrenheit and in Celsius) it would be very unlikely to have a situation where two variables are exactly correlated with one another. A more likely scenario is to have variables that are not sufficiently different for the model to distinguish them. For example, Phibbs and colleagues found that birth weight and gestational age were too closely related to include both in their analysis of neonatal mortality.[2]

If you include two or more variables that are multicollinear, the coefficients (Section 8.3) of the variables will be unstable: they will likely have very large standard errors and wide confidence intervals. You will not be able to accurately judge the importance of the individual variables to the outcome. However, the overall model will still be accurate. In fact one clue of potential multicollinearity is that the overall model is statistically significant even though the individual coefficients are not.[3]

5.2 How do I assess whether my variables are multicollinear?

The correlation coefficient (also called Pearson correlation coefficient or r) is a bivariate statistic that measures how strongly two variables are related to one another. The correlation coefficient assumes the relationship between the two variables is linear. It can range from –1 to 1. When the coefficient is –1 or 1 the two variables change together exactly (i.e., knowing one variable tells you the value of the other variable). The only difference between –1 and 1 is that the negative sign indicates that the two variables change exactly together in opposite directions (i.e., as one goes higher the other goes lower). Zero indicates that there is no relationship whatsoever. If you square the correlation coefficient and multiply by 100 you get a measure of how much information the two variables share ranging from 0 percent to 100 percent.

The correlation between temperature in Fahrenheit and in Celsius is 1.0. The two variables share 100 percent of the same information. In contrast, the correlation between vitamin B_{12} level and pneumococcal antibody titer following immunization was found to be 0.61 (Figure 3.1). The two variables share 37 percent ($0.61^2 \times 100 = 37$) of the same information.

---

[2] Phibbs, C. S., Bronstein, J. M., Buston, W., *et al.* "The effects of patient volume and level of care at the hospital of birth on neonatal mortality." *JAMA* **276** (1996): 1054–9.

[3] Computing Center at University of Kentucky. "Multicollinearity in Logistic Regression" available at http://www.uky.edu/ComputingCenter/SSTARS/MulticollinearityinLogisticRegression.htm.

To determine how correlated your independent variables are you may run a correlation coefficient matrix with all your proposed independent variables. In general, two variables that are correlated at more than 0.90 will pose problems in your analysis. Variables correlated at 0.80 or more may also pose problems. Unfortunately, even if all the correlations in the matrix are less than 0.80 this is no guarantee that you will not have problems with multicollinearity.

A major reason that the correlation matrix is inadequate for assessing whether you will have problems owing to multicollinearity is that a correlation matrix only provides information on the relationship between two variables. However it is equally problematic – but harder to diagnose – when you have three or more independent variables that are highly related to one another. In a sense we have already dealt with this concept in Section 4.2 on converting nominal variables into multiple dichotomous variables ("dummy variables"). Look back at Table 4.1. You will recall that I said you did not need to create a variable for white ethnicity because if a subject were 0 (no) on the variables for African-American, Latino/Hispanic, Asian/Pacific Islander, Native American, and other nonwhite ethnicity the subject would be of white ethnicity. What if you didn't read this section and entered into your model a yes/no variable for each ethnicity including white? Then you would have a situation where a combination of independent variables completely accounts for the value of a different independent variable. Prove this to yourself, by correctly answering the following questions:

1. A subject is "yes" on any one of the five variables: African-American, Latino/Hispanic, Asian/Pacific Islander, Native American, or other nonwhite ethnicity. What is the subject's value on the white ethnicity variable?
2. A different subject is "no" on all five of the variables: African-American, Latino/Hispanic, Asian/Pacific Islander, Native American, or other nonwhite ethnicity. What is the subject's value on the white ethnicity variable?

You knew that the answer to the first question was **No** and the answer to the second question was **Yes**, even though I didn't tell you anything about the subject's value on the variable of white ethnicity. This is a situation where a combination of variables completely determines the value of another variable. If you entered a variable for white ethnicity, in addition to the others, this would result in spurious results in your multivariable model.

How will you know if a combination of variables accounts for another variable's value? Two related measures of multicollinearity are tolerance and the reciprocal of tolerance: the variance inflation factor. Both measure how much the regression coefficient for a particular variable is determined by the other independent variables in the model.

TIP

Two variables correlated at > 0.8 may cause multicollinearity problems in your analysis.

Because multicollinearity concerns the relationship of the independent variables to each other, rather than the relationship of the independent variables to the dependent variables, the calculation of these two measures of multicollinearity does not vary based on the type of multivariable analysis you will be performing. You may find that these statistics are calculated within the linear regression section of your computerized statistical software packages. Go ahead and use the routines within linear regression even if you will be performing a logistic, proportional hazards, or Poisson regression analysis, since neither the outcome variable nor the method of multivariable analysis changes the calculation of these statistics.

There are no hard and fast rules about what cut-offs of these statistics indicate a degree of multicollinearity that would jeopardize the validity of your analysis. In general, small tolerance values, including those below 0.25, are worrisome, and those below 0.10 are serious. As you would expect with a reciprocal value, it is high values of the variance inflation factor that indicate multicollinearity. Variance inflation factors greater than 2.5 may be problematic, whereas values greater than ten are serious.[4]

If the values of some of your variables are worrisome, you will need to do additional analyses to determine which of the other variables in the model are closely related with the problematic variable. This can be done by performing regression analyses using the other variables as independent variables to estimate the value of the problematic variable. This will show you which variables are highly related and enable you to decide which variables to keep in the analysis.

Besides the situation where the overall model is statistically significant but none of the predictors are (Section 5.1), another clue that you may have a problem with multicollinearity is when addition or deletion of a variable causes substantial changes in the coefficients of the other variables.

> **TIP**
>
> Use the routines in the linear regression program for calculating tolerance and variance inflation factor even if you are performing a different kind of multivariable model.

> **TIP**
>
> When addition or deletion of a variable from a model causes substantial changes in the coefficients of other variables, consider that you may have problems owing to multicollinearity.

5.3 What should I do with multicollinear variables?

If you have variables that are highly related, consider your options:

- omit the variable
- use an "and/or" clause, or
- create a scale

---

[4] For more on measures of multicollinearity and when to worry, see: Glantz, S.A. and Slinker, B.K. *Primer of Applied Regression and Analysis of Variance.* New York, NY: McGraw-Hill, 1990, pp. 181–99.

If you are going to omit one of the variables, how do you decide which one to delete? Omit the one that is theoretically less important, has more missing data, has more measurement error, or is less satisfactory in some other way. In the study of neonatal mortality referred to above, the investigators kept birth weight and excluded gestational age. They excluded gestational age because there were more missing cases on this variable than on birth weight and it was less reliably coded. Ironically, as the authors point out, gestational age is theoretically the more important factor in accounting for mortality (because age, not weight, is the deciding factor in reaching certain fetal developmental milestones). Therefore they included two additional variables in their analysis (small for gestational age [yes/no] and large for gestational age [yes/no]) to adjust for the fact that weight might not be an accurate measure of gestational age in some cases.

> **TIP**
>
> If you need to omit a variable, omit the one that has more missing data, has more measurement error, or is less satisfactory in some other way.

Using "and/or" clauses works well for correlated variables that represent the same process. For example, if you asked patients with pneumonia whether they had diaphoresis (sweats) or rigors (shaking), these two variables would be expected to be closely correlated since rigors are a more extreme form of diaphoresis. However, some patients who had rigors may not have noticed that they were first diaphoretic; some who were diaphoretic may have taken aspirin thereby preventing the rigor. The new variable could be diaphoresis and/or rigor. Patients who had one or both would be reported as "yes" on this variable; those who had neither would be reported as "no."

Creating multi-item scales is a strategy often pursued with psychological and sociologic data. In creating scales, the values of multiple variables for each subject are summated or averaged to form a single variable that summarizes the meaning of the separate variables (Section 6.5.C.3). Researchers may intentionally ask subjects multiple related questions to test the reliability of the subject's responses (i.e., when asked a similar question, using different wording, will subjects answer in the same way?). In this case, researchers usually plan ahead of time which questions will form a scale. Other times researchers will use factor analysis (Section 6.5.C.4) to determine which questions provide similar information.

These techniques for dealing with multicollinear variables also work when you need to decrease the number of independent variables in your analysis because of insufficient sample size. However, they will not work for decreasing sample size if your variables are not highly related. A variety of methods for decreasing the number of independent variables are detailed in Section 6.5.

Setting up a multivariable analysis

6.1 What independent variables should I include in my multivariable model?

On the surface this seems like a simple question. You should include the risk factor(s) of interest and any variables that may potentially confound the relationship between the risk factor and the outcome. However deciding which variables may confound your analysis is not always easy. Variables that are extraneous, redundant, have a lot of missing data, or intervene between your risk factor and outcome should be excluded.

Recommendations on what variables to include and exclude in your model are reviewed in Table 6.1 and discussed in the next two sections.

6.2 How do I decide what confounders to include in my model?

> **TIP**
>
> Include in your model those variables that have been theorized or shown in prior research to be confounders of the relationship you are studying.

Ideally researchers should include all those variables that have been theorized or shown in prior research to be confounders. Depending on the outcome you are studying, there may be a large number of variables that have been shown in prior research to be associated with the risk factor and the outcome. For example, studies of cardiovascular outcomes must include a large number of potential outcomes including age, sex, smoking status, hypertension, diabetes, obesity, LDL-cholesterol, HDL-cholesterol, reactive C-protein, aspirin use, and beta-blocker use because all of these variables have already been shown to affect cardiovascular disease.

In addition to including variables that have been theorized or shown in prior research to be confounders, include in your model those variables that fit the empiric definition of confounders in your data. Specifically, include those independent variables that are associated with the risk factor and the outcome in bivariate analysis, unless you believe that those variables are intervening between the risk factor and the outcome (Section 6.3).

Unfortunately, there is no single standard of how strong an association should be to result in a variable being included as a potential confounder.

TIP

Include in your models those variables that are associated with the risk factor and the outcome in bivariate analysis.

In general, you want to err on the side of inclusion. Most investigators will include in their multivariable model any variable that is associated with the outcome at a P value of < 0.20 or 0.25, regardless of whether or not the variable has been shown to be associated with the risk factor. (In using empiric criteria for choosing variables to enter into your multivariable analysis, keep in mind that if you have a suppresser effect, the variable may not be even weakly associated with the outcome in bivariate analysis. Recall the example in Section 1.3 of zidovudine treatment, which affected the likelihood of seroconversion in multivariable analysis even though it was not significantly related to seroconversion in bivariate analysis.)

Remember that even if you use an empiric criterion to decide which variables to enter into your model, you should still include those that are theoretically important or have been confounders in prior research even if they did not meet your criterion. For example, Spencer and colleagues in their study of the effectiveness of statin therapy in patients with acute coronary syndrome (described in Section 2.3) included in their multivariable models variables that were associated with the outcome of interest in bivariate analysis at a P value of < 0.25.[1] They then used a stepwise model (Section 7.8) to exclude variables that were not associated with the outcome at a P value of ≤ 0.05. However, they included age, sex, and history of hyperlipidemia in all final models regardless of their statistical significance because of their clinical relevance to coronary artery syndromes.

6.3 What independent variables should I exclude from my multivariable model?

In building accurate models, what variables you exclude is as important as what variables you include (Table 6.1). Exclude from your multivariable model extraneous variables, i.e., variables that are not on the causal pathway to your outcome. For example, if you are developing a model estimating HIV prevalence, and you are using the large multipurpose National Health and Nutrition Examination Survey (NHANES), exclude from your model seat-belt use, even though it may well be associated with safer-sex practices (because people who are health conscious are likely to use both seat belts and condoms). Because seat-belt use is not on the causal pathway between behavior and HIV infection, including it can only add error to your model (since all measurements have error) and confusion to your readers.

---

[1] Spencer, F. A., Allegrone, J., Goldberg, R. J., *et al.* "Association of statin therapy with outcomes of acute coronary syndromes: The Grace study." *Ann. Intern. Med.* **140** (2004): 857–66.

Table 6.1 Variables to include and exclude in multivariable models.

What to include?	What to exclude?
Risk factor(s)	Extraneous variables (variables not on the causal pathway to your outcome)
Potential confounders, based on theory, prior research, empirical findings	Redundant variables
	Variables with a lot of missing data
	Intervening variables (variables that are on the causal pathway between a risk factor and an outcome)

It is also important to exclude redundant variables. The strength of multivariable analysis is that it can determine the unique contribution of related variables to outcome. However, if two variables are too closely related, multivariable analysis cannot accurately separate the impact of the two variables on outcome. This problem is called multicollinearity (Chapter 5) and requires that you enter only one of the highly related variables. For example, in a study of factors associated with adherence to combination antiretroviral medication among HIV-infected persons, the investigators found that ethnicity was collinear with acculturation; they chose to put ethnicity in the model and exclude acculturation.[2]

> With duplicative variables include the one that is theoretically more important, has less missing data, or has less measurement error.

When deciding which of two duplicative variables to include, choose the one that is theoretically more important, has less missing data, or has less measurement error.

It is also important to exclude variables with a lot of missing data. Missing data is a much greater problem with multivariable analysis than bivariate analysis. This is because subjects with missing values on any of the variables entered into the model are tossed out of the analysis even if the subject has valid values on the other variables. (With a bivariate analysis, you lose only those subjects with missing values on the two variables used, not those with missing values on the other variables.)

> **TIP**
> Drop variables rather than subjects when you have missing data.

Dropped subjects decrease the power of your analysis and, perhaps even more problematically, bias your study because subjects missing on a particular variable may be systematically different than subjects not missing on that variable. Because it is generally better to lose variables than subjects, drop variables that have a lot of missing data.

That being said, sometimes you have a variable of such great importance that it must be included in your analysis even if there are many missing cases.

---

[2] Golin, C. E., Liu, H., Hays, R. D., *et al.* "A prospective study of predictors of adherence to combination antiretroviral medication." *J. Gen. Intern. Med.* **17** (2002): 756–65.

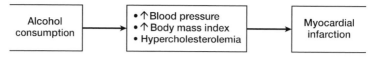

Figure 6.1

HDL is an intervening variable between moderate alcohol consumption and decreased coronary artery disease.

If this is the case, acknowledge to your readers that the missing cases may bias your results in ways that are hard to assess. You can provide some reassurance to your readers if a comparison of cases with missing data to cases without missing data shows no difference on important characteristics. Alternatively, you may use one of the available methods for assigning values to missing cases, thereby enabling you to use the variable in the analysis (Section 6.6).

You should also exclude variables that are on the causal pathway to your outcome. Such variables are referred to as intervening variables. It may seem confusing that I recommend excluding intervening variables since I said earlier that you should exclude variables *not* on the causal pathway to your outcome. Why am I now telling you to exclude variables that are on the causal pathway?

The reason is that if you statistically adjust for an intervening variable, you may adjust away the very effect you are trying to demonstrate. For example, it is known that moderate alcohol consumption is associated with a lower incidence of coronary artery disease. The mechanism appears to be that moderate alcohol consumption increases the HDL-cholesterol, the "good cholesterol" as shown in Figure 6.1.

If you adjust for HDL level in an analysis of the effect of alcohol consumption on coronary artery disease, it may appear that alcohol has no effect. However, that's not accurate; alcohol use is causally related to coronary heart disease, but the effect is mediated by HDL-cholesterol. This problem is referred to as overadjustment.[3]

Unfortunately there is no test for whether a variable is a confounder or an intervening variable. Statistically confounders and intervening variables act the same. Therefore the decision on whether to include a variable in a model because you believe it is a confounder, or exclude it because you believe it is an intervening variable, should be made based on prior research and biological plausibility.

One circumstance in which it is appropriate to include an intervening variable is if you are trying to demonstrate that the effect of a risk factor on outcome

DEFINITION

An intervening variable is on the causal pathway to your outcome.

TIP

Don't adjust for an intervening variable or you may adjust away the effect you are trying to demonstrate.

TIP

Statistically confounders and intervening variables act the same.

---

[3] Szklo. M. and Nieto, F. J. *Epidemiology: Beyond the Basics.* Gaithersburg: Aspen Publishers, 2000, p. 333.

is mediated by an intervening variable. In such cases, you will want to run the model first without the intervening variable and then a second time with the intervening variable. If it is an intervening variable, the statistical association between the risk factor and the outcome seen in the first model will be eliminated or dampened in the second model. This can be helpful in understanding the mechanism by which a risk factor affects the outcome. (But keep in mind that the association between risk factor and outcome will also diminish with inclusion of a confounding variable.)

6.4 How many subjects do I need to do multivariable analysis?

TIP

The smaller the effect, the larger the sample size needed to demonstrate a statistically significant effect.

TIP

The more variability there is in your measures the larger the sample size needed to demonstrate a statistically significant effect.

DEFINITION

A *power* calculation determines the needed sample size to detect a particular effect.

TIP

If your power calculation shows that you do not have enough subjects for demonstrating the effect in bivariate analysis, you definitely will not have enough subjects to demonstrate the effect in multivariable analysis.

The sample size needed for multivariable analysis, as with bivariate analysis, depends on the size of the effect you are trying to demonstrate and the variability of the data. It takes a much larger sample size to show that a risk factor is mildly (but statistically) associated with an outcome (e.g., odds ratio of 1.5) than to show that it is strongly associated with an outcome (e.g., odds ratio of 4.0). The reason is that the smaller the sample size, the larger the confidence intervals. The closer the odds ratio is to 1.0 then the more likely wide confidence intervals are to include one. Similarly, although you can never prove the null hypothesis (i.e., no association: odds ratio of 1.0), the larger the sample size the smaller the chance that you have missed an association that was really present. It also takes a larger sample size to demonstrate a difference between groups on a variable that has a great deal of variability (i.e., a large standard deviation).

Determining the needed sample size is referred to as a power calculation (the power to detect a result). Power calculations for multivariable analysis are complicated and generally require consultation with a biostatistician. However, as a start, determine the sample size needed for a bivariate analysis (i.e., a comparison of two proportions, a comparison of two means, a comparison of two times to outcome without adjustment for other variables). Several free and easy-to-use computer software programs exist to do this.[4] If your power calculation shows that you do not have enough subjects to demonstrate the effect in bivariate analysis, you definitely will not have enough subjects in your

---

[4] Free software packages for doing sample size calculations are available: Statistical Considerations for Clinical Trials and Scientific Experiments by David Schoenfeld (http://hedwig.mgh. harvard.edu/sample_size/quan_measur/defs.html) and Simple Interactive Statistical Analysis (SISA) (http://home.clara.net/sisa/sampshlp.htm). See: Katz, M.H. *Study Design and Statistical Analysis: A Practical Guide for Clinicians.* Cambridge University Press, 2006, Chapter 7, for explanations of the needed ingredients to input into these computer programs. Alternatively, for an easy-to-follow sample-size guide that doesn't require computer software, see: Hulley, S.B., Cummings, S.R., Browner, W.S., *et al. Designing Clinical Research* (2nd edn). Baltimore, MD: Lippincott Williams and Wilkins, 2001, pp. 65–91.

multivariable analysis. If it shows that you do have enough subjects, the next question would be whether the sample size is sufficient for your multivariable analysis.

For those ready to go to the next level, the easiest way to perform a multivariable sample-size calculation is to use an available software program. Power and Precision (http://www.power-analysis.com/specifications.htm) calculates the needed sample size for multiple linear regression and multiple logistic regression. The NCSS Statistical and Power Analysis Softwear (PASS) program (http://www.ncss.com) calculates the needed sample size for multiple linear regression, multiple logistic regression, proportional hazards analysis, and Poisson regression. Both have free trial periods. Although the programs are easy to use, I strongly advise having a biostatistician check your assumptions if you have not done sample-size calculations for multivariable analysis previously.

For all of the sample-size calculations you will need to state the alpha (usually 0.05 and two-tailed) and the beta (usually 0.80).

To compute the needed sample size for a multiple linear regression design using the Power and Precision program you need to specify the number of variables that represent your hypothesis (i.e., the risk factor[s]) and the number of variables that are covariates (i.e., the set of potential confounders). For the set of risk factor(s) and the set of covariates you need to specify the increment of R^2 (Section 8.2.A) that you anticipate that each set will explain. The program will also allow you to calculate the needed sample size for more complicated models (e.g., a linear regression model with an interaction term, a linear regression model with a risk factor, the square of the value of the risk factor, and a cubic transformation of the value of the risk factor).

The PASS program uses different parameters than Power and Precision for calculating the sample size for multiple linear regression. Specifically, you will need to enter the slope assuming the null hypothesis, the slope assuming the alternative hypothesis, the standard deviation of the independent variables, and the standard deviation of the dependent variable (the latter is needed in addition to the slope of the alternative hypothesis, and the standard deviation of the independent variables, for calculating the standard deviation of the residuals; the package also offers an alternative method for calculating the standard deviation of the residuals.)

To calculate sample size for logistic regression with a dichotomous independent variable using Power and Precision, you will need to specify the relative proportion in each group (e.g., 1:1 if equal numbers of subjects in each group; 2:1 if twice the number in one group as the other). A convenient feature of Power and Precision is that it will allow you to enter a categorical variable (e.g., ethnicity in four categories) and it will automatically create multiple dichotomous variables with a reference category, so that you can determine the needed sample size for a logistic regression model with a categorical independent variable.

To calculate sample size for multiple logistic regression with an interval-independent variable you will need to specify the mean and standard deviation of the independent variable, the event rate at the mean (the event rate at the mean is the same for all variables), and the event rate at a point other than the mean for the independent variable. The program Power and Precision can accomodate two interval-independent variables. If you include two you will need to specify the correlation between them (with the correct sign).

To calculate sample size for multiple logistic regression using the PASS program, you will need to specify the baseline probability (the probability of outcome when the dichotomous covariates equal 0 or if you have interval covariates when they are equal to the mean), the expected odds ratio, the R^2 when the independent variable of interest is regressed on the other independent variables in the regression (i.e., the independent variable of interest is used as the dependent variable in a regression design where the other independent variables are used to predict it).

To calculate sample size with proportional hazards analysis, you can use the PASS program. You will need to specify the event rate, which is the proportion of noncensored subjects in whom the outcome occurs during the duration of the study. You will also need to specify the natural log of the expected hazard ratio, and the R^2 when the independent variable of interest is regressed on the other independent variables in the regression (i.e., independent variable of interest is used as the dependent variable in a regression design where the other independent variables are used to predict it).

To calculate the needed sample size for Poisson analysis using PASS, you will need to specify the baseline response rate, the response rate ratio (the response rate owing to a one-unit change in the independent variable divided by the baseline response), the mean exposure time, the phi (overdispersion parameter) of the response, and the R^2 when the independent variable of interest is regressed on the other independent variables in the regression (i.e., independent variable of interest is used as the dependent variable in a regression design where the other independent variables are used to predict it.).

Although not an alternative to formally calculating the needed sample size, a useful rule-of-thumb for planning multiple logistic regression and proportional hazards analysis is that for every independent variable in your model

TIP

For multiple logistic regression and proportional hazards analysis you should have at least ten outcomes for each independent variable in your model.

you need at least ten outcomes.[5] The reason I say ten outcomes for each independent variable, rather than 20 subjects for each independent variable (which would be equivalent if your outcome occurred in half your subjects), is that your model is assessing a particular outcome. In most medical studies, less than half of the subjects experience the outcome (e.g., develop cancer or have a heart attack). If your outcome occurs in only five subjects in your study you may not have enough power to answer your research question even if you have a thousand other subjects in whom the outcome does not occur. This is because the model is determining the likelihood of outcome based on those five people. It does not help you to determine the likelihood of no outcome if this is the larger group. The needed sample size is based on the smaller of the two groups. The reason is that outcome and not outcome are mathematically equivalent: the likelihood of not outcome is simply 1 – (the likelihood of outcome).

The ten outcomes per variable is just a guideline. Just because your sample size does not meet this criterion does not mean that your study won't appear in the *New England Journal of Medicine* (see Chambers and colleagues, example in Section 6.5.A). Conversely, even if you have ten outcomes for each independent variable you still may not have an adequate sample size to answer your study question. For example, you may not have enough subjects in one of the categories of a dichotomous independent variable to study its association with outcome. Just as the sample size depends on the less common outcome state, the sample size to demonstrate that a particular independent variable is associated with your outcome will depend on the less common of the values of the dichotomous independent variable.

An example will help to illustrate this principle. Schwarcz and colleagues performed a logistic regression analysis to assess the factors associated with having received pneumocystis prophylaxis prior to a diagnosis of pneumocystis pneumonia (PCP) among HIV-infected persons.[6] The total sample size was 326 persons diagnosed with PCP. Of these, 114 (35 percent) had received prophylaxis prior to their diagnosis of PCP and 212 (65 percent) had not. The model included six independent variables. Since the smaller group (those who

[5] Peduzzi, P., Concato, J., Kemper, E., *et al.* "A simulation study of the number of events per variable in logistic regression analysis." *J. Clin. Epidemiol.* **49** (1996): 1373–9; Peduzzi, P., Concato, J., Feinstein, A. R., *et al.* "Importance of events per independent variable in proportional hazards regression analysis II. Accuracy and precision of regression estimates." *J. Clin. Epidemiol.* **48** (1995): 1503–10; Harrell, F. E., Lee, K. L., Matchar, D. B., *et al.* "Regression models for prognostic prediction: Advantages, problems, and suggested solutions." *Cancer Treat. Rep.* **69** (1985): 1071–7.
[6] Schwarcz, S. K., Katz, M. H., Hirozawa, A., *et al.* "Prevention of *Pneumocystis carinii* pneumonia: Who are we missing?" *AIDS* **11** (1997): 1263–8.

Table 6.2 Frequency of primary PCP prophylaxis among patients whose AIDS-defining diagnosis was PCP.

Characteristic	Did not receive PCP prophylaxis n (%)	Received primary PCP prophylaxis n (%)	Adjusted P value	Adjusted odds ratio	95% confidence limits
Total	212 (65.0)	114 (35.0)			
Age group					
< 35 years	61 (69.3)	27 (30.7)		1.0 (ref.)	
≥ 35 years	151 (63.5)	87 (36.6)	0.55	1.19	0.68, 2.07
Ethnicity					
Nonwhite	74 (77.9)	21 (22.1)		0.49	0.28, 0.87
White	138 (59.7)	93 (40.3)	0.01	1.0 (ref.)	
Sex					
Male	206 (64.6)	113 (35.4)		0.81	0.06, 10.12
Female	6 (85.7)	1 (14.3)	0.87	1.0 (ref.)	
Sexual orientation					
Gay/bisexual man	185 (62.7)	110 (37.3)		3.19	0.78, 13.03
Heterosexual	27 (87.1)	4 (12.9)	0.11	1.0 (ref.)	
Injection drug use					
Yes	35 (72.9)	13 (27.1)		1.11	0.49, 2.54
No	177 (63.7)	101 (36.3)	0.80	1.0 (ref.)	
Insurance					
None	52 (82.5)	11 (17.5)		0.35	0.17, 0.73
Public/private	151 (59.5)	103 (40.6)	0.005	1.0 (ref.)	

Adapted with permission from Schwarcz, S. K., *et al.* "Prevention of *Pneumocystis carinii* pneumonia: Who are we missing?" *AIDS* **11** (1997): 1263–8. Copyright Rapid Science Publishers Ltd.

had received prophylaxis) was 114 there would appear to be enough subjects; using our rule of thumb we would need only 60 subjects in the smaller group.

As you can see in Table 6.2, two variables were significantly associated (adjusted *P* value < 0.05) with a lower likelihood of having received prophylaxis in the logistic regression analysis: being nonwhite and being uninsured. Note that the confidence intervals for these two variables exclude one and are reasonably narrow.

Gender was not significantly associated with receipt of prophylaxis: The odds ratio was 0.81. However, before concluding that the study showed that gender was not important, one must note that the 95 percent confidence intervals for gender were 0.06 to 10.12. In other words, it is equally likely that women are a sixteenth as likely or ten times more likely to receive prophylaxis. Obviously, this result is of little scientific value. The study only had seven women (2 percent of sample); the model had little information on which to base an estimate of the likelihood of having received prophylaxis for this group and this is reflected in a large standard error and a broad confidence interval. A similar situation can be seen for the variable of sexual orientation. Because there were only 31 heterosexuals (10 percent of sample), the confidence intervals for the risk estimate associated with sexual orientation were very broad: 0.78 to 13.03.

In general, large standard errors and large confidence intervals (which are based on standard errors) are clues of an inadequate sample size. Another, more dramatic indication that you do not have a large enough sample size in logistic regression, proportional hazards analysis, and Poisson regression is if the model does not converge. There is simply not enough information, usually because of too few outcomes, for the computer to solve the equation. Although you can increase the number of attempts the computer makes to solve the equation if your model fails to converge, you should consider the possibility that you do not have enough subjects to answer your research question.

> **TIP**
>
> For multiple linear regression you should have 20 subjects for each independent variable in your model.

For multiple linear regression 20 subjects (rather than outcome events) per independent variable is recommended.[7] The reason that the sample size rule of thumb for multiple linear regression is based on study subjects rather than numbers of outcome as with logistic regression and proportional hazards regression is that with linear regression you can consider all subjects as having experienced the outcome (because the outcome is interval). However, just as with these other techniques you will have very large standard errors (and therefore large confidence intervals) if you do not have a large enough sample size. Although this is a very reasonable standard, it does not mean that all analyses with fewer subjects are invalid; you just need to show more caution in interpreting the coefficients.

The formulae for calculating sample size for Poisson regression for both bivariate and multivariable analyses are also available.[8]

6.5 What if I have too many independent variables given my sample size?

If your power calculations or analyses show you have too many independent variables for your sample size, you need to increase the number of subjects or decrease the number of independent variables. Although increasing the number of subjects is more desirable, it is usually impossible in the analysis

---

[7] Feinstein, A. R. *Multivariable Analysis: An Introduction*. New Haven: Yale University Press, 1996, p. 226.
[8] Signorini, D. F. "Sample size for Poisson regression." *Biometrika* **78** (1991): 446–50.

Table 6.3 Methods for decreasing the number of independent variables.

---

1. Exclude variables that are not empirically operating as confounders.

    Variable unrelated to main independent variable and outcome in bivariate
      analysis

    Variable has minimal impact on main effect in multivariable analysis

    Variable excluded by variable selection algorithm

2. Choose one variable to represent two or more related variables.

3. Combine variables into a single variable, score or scale.

    "And/or" constructions

    Scores

    Multi-item scales

    Factor analysis

---

phase. Most researchers will therefore attempt to reduce the number of independent variables in their analysis.

For example, let's say you have determined from Sections 6.1–6.2 that you would like to include 20 independent variables in your multivariable model but your sample size is sufficient for inclusion of only ten variables. What should you do?

Assuming that you have already excluded extraneous variables, redundant variables, variables with a lot of missing data, and intervening variables (Table 6.1), then you will need additional options. Other methods for reducing the number of variables in your model are shown in Table 6.3.

6.5.A   Exclude variables that are not empirically operating as confounders

In Section 6.2, I explained that it is best, where possible, to use an inclusive definition of potential confounders, so as to lessen the chance that you are missing subtle forms of confounding (e.g., several weakly associated variables may together have a substantial impact on the main effect).

However, when you do not have a sufficient sample size you must set more stringent criteria for inclusion of variables in your model. For example, you may want to include only those variables that are associated with both the independent variable of interest and the outcome variable in bivariate analyses. Remember, unless both of these conditions are met, the variable cannot be a confounder or a suppresser.

A variation of this strategy is to include only those independent variables that change the size of your main effect by a predetermined amount. For example, Chambers and colleagues studied whether fluoxetine (Prozac) affected birth outcomes.[9] They compared the rate of prematurity among 98 infants whose mothers had taken fluoxetine early in pregnancy only to 70 infants whose mothers had taken it late in pregnancy. Only 14 infants were born prematurely. To limit the number of variables in the model, they included only those independent variables that changed the estimate of the main effect (early-only versus late exposure to fluoxetine on prematurity) by more than ten percent. Eleven variables met this criterion and were included in the model, in addition to two other variables (maternal age and dose of fluoxetine), which were included for theoretical reasons.

With a total of 13 independent variables and only 14 outcomes, the investigators were far from fulfilling the guideline of ten outcomes per variable. Late exposure to fluoxetine was associated with an increased risk of prematurity: odds ratio of 4.8. Reflecting the relatively small number of outcomes and the large number of independent variables, the 95 percent confidence intervals for the effect of fluoxetine on prematurity were large, ranging from 1.1 to 20.8. Because the confidence intervals excluded one, the data suggest that late exposure to fluoxetine is associated with an increased risk of prematurity. However, in weighing the benefits versus risks, there is a large difference between an odds ratio of 1.1 and one of 20.8.

Variable selection algorithms (statistical procedures used to select which of your independent variables to include or keep in your multivariable model) are also used to deal with small sample sizes. However, these procedures have substantial drawbacks (Section 7.8).

6.5.B   Choose one variable to represent two or more related variables

When you have two or more variables that are *moderately* correlated with one another, you may want to choose one to enter into your model to jointly represent the others. (I have italicized moderately as a reminder that we are not talking about variables that are multicollinear [Sections 5.1–5.3].) For example, income, education, and job status are correlated in the United States, but not to a degree that they would usually cause problems with multicollinearity. Ideally, in an analysis where it was important to adjust for socioeconomic status you would include all three variables. However, if this were impossible because of inadequate sample size, then including one would partially adjust your analyses for socioeconomic status. When variables are correlated, by including one, you include some of the information from the other variables. However, unless they are perfectly correlated, you will lose potentially important information

---

[9] Chambers, C. D., Johnson, K. A., Dick, L. M., *et al.* "Birth outcomes in pregnant women taking fluoxetine." *New. Engl. J. Med.* **335** (1996): 1010–15.

by excluding one or more. The amount of information lost depends on the degree of correlation. In terms of the decision as to which variable to keep and which to exclude, the decision-making process is the same as with multicollinearity. Keep the variable that is theoretically superior, has less missing data, or has less measurement error. When available, a better solution than choosing one variable to represent a set of variables is to construct a score or scale to represent a group of variables (see next section).

6.5.C   Methods of combining multiple variables into a single variable, score or scale

Sometimes you can reduce the number of independent variables in your analysis without omitting a variable. This is done by combining variables into a single variable. Four methods are commonly used: "and/or" constructions, scores, multi-item scales, and factor analysis.

6.5.C.1 Use of "and/or" constructions

Two or more related variables can be combined with the use of an "and/or" clause (Section 5.3). For example, in the study of the effect of perinatal exposure to fluoxetine on birth outcomes, the investigators combined hypertension, pre-eclampsia, and eclampsia as one variable. In other words, women who suffered from hypertension, pre-eclampsia, eclampsia, or more than one of the three, would be "yes" on the variable; women who had none of these conditions would be "no." This fits the pathophysiology in that the three conditions are progressive states of the same underlying condition. And/or clauses may also be helpful when you have variables that are multicollinear (all women with eclampsia by definition have pre-eclampsia) or when you have an independent variable with almost everyone in the same group (as you would if you had a variable of eclampsia yes/no – almost everyone would be no, since eclampsia is relatively rare). Independent variables where almost everyone is in the same group tend to have large standard errors and large confidence intervals.

6.5.C.2 Scores

One straightforward method of reducing the number of independent variables is simply to score the number of risk factors for the disease that each subject has. For example, Turner and Lloyd computed a score to measure the lifetime exposure to adversity.[10] Subjects were assessed as to whether they had been

[10] Turner, R. J. and Lloyd, D. A. "Stress burden and the lifetime incidence of psychiatric disorder in young adults." *Arch. Gen. Psych.* **61** (2004): 481–8.

exposed to 33 adverse life events (e.g., failing a grade in school, losing a home due to a natural disaster, being physically abused or injured). The number of adverse events experienced was totaled (i.e., the score could range from 0 to 33). The investigators found that higher scores were associated with an increased risk of developing a depressive and/or anxiety disorder.

6.5.C.3 Multi-item scales

Investigators may use scales (sets of closely related questions) to measure constructs that are difficult to assess by a single question (e.g., attitudes, treatment preferences). The decision to create a scale is usually made in the design phase, although researchers sometimes find, in the analytic phase, that a group of variables measure a reliable construct.

To create a scale, first code all questions in the same direction, so that, for example, a higher score is better on all items. You must also recode variables so that they are all on the same numeric scales. Otherwise variables measured on a 0 to 10 scale will have twice the weight in the total score as variables measured on a 0 to 5 scale. Dividing a 0 to 10 scale by two will put it on the same scale as a 0 to 5 scale. You can then summate the items or average them by dividing the sum by the number of variables in the scale. In creating scales you must pay close attention to the handling of missing data on individual items. If, for a particular subject, the majority of items that constitute the scale have missing values then the value for the scale should be missing for that subject. If at least half of the items, for a particular subject, have a valid response, you can replace the missing values with the mean for the sample on the particular items that are missing. Once you have replaced the missing values, you can then summate the scale and divide by the number of variables in the scale.

There is an alternative method for handling missing cases when constructing scales. You can compute the average for each subject by dividing the total by the number of variables for which the subject has valid responses. For example, if a particular subject had valid responses for four of the five variables that constitute a scale, you could summate their four questions and divide by four. In comparison, for subjects with complete values, you would summate their five questions and divide by five. If you are using this technique, at least half of the variables that constitute the scale for each subject must have complete data. Assign a missing value to subjects who have more than half the variables with missing data. (Some would assign a missing value only if a fourth or more of the questions have missing responses.)[11]

---

[11] Hull, C. H. and Nie, N. H. *SPSS Update 7–9*. New York, NY: McGraw-Hill, 1989, p. 257.

This type of multi-item scale will work only if the variables are highly correlated. The usual measure of how correlated the variables are to one another is the alpha (also referred to as a reliability coefficient). Alphas greater than 0.65 generally indicate that the variables form a reliable scale. To achieve alphas of this level, the questions are usually written with the intention of scoring them together.

The biggest difference between scales and scores is this requirement that scales use related questions. In the case of a score, the items do not need to be related. Using the example of the lifetime exposure to adversity score discussed above, failing a grade in school and witnessing a natural disaster would not be expected to be highly correlated, but are both certainly significant life stresses.

6.5.C.4 Factor analysis

Factor analysis is a popular strategy in the behavioral sciences for reducing the number of variables in cases where you have multiple related independent variables. Factor analysis summarizes multiple related independent variables (say 15) into a few underlying factors (say two or three). The procedure minimizes the correlations between the factors (so that they represent distinct dimensions). Each factor is a weighted combination of the original variables. As such you can develop a factor score for each subject based on that subject's values for each of the variables, thereby reducing the number of variables to the number of factors. Each of the independent variables will be correlated with each of the factors, but to varying degrees. For any one of the factors, a few of the variables will be strongly correlated with it, indicating that the factor primarily represents this cluster of variables. Based on these correlations (referred to as loadings) you can characterize the nature of the factor (i.e., what it represents).

The major problem with factor analysis for clinical researchers is the loss of the original variables. Let's say, for example, you used factor analysis to develop factor scores for variables associated with survival from pneumonia. Assume the first factor was characterized by patient comorbidity (age, underlying lung disease, history of congestive heart failure), the second factor was characterized by virulence of attack (severity of radiological findings, peak of fever, specific organism recovered), and the third factor was characterized by efficacy of treatment (speed of first dose, appropriate choice of antibiotics). This would be a very satisfying characterization of the data from the point of view of the pathophysiology of pneumonia.

Assume that a proportional hazards model demonstrates that the factors of patient co-morbidity and virulence of attack are associated with a worse survival, whereas efficacious treatment is associated with an improved survival. How useful would these results be to a clinician? Certainly, clinicians could not use the information to generate a probability of survival for their patients because it would be mathematically too complicated to generate factor scores. Also, you couldn't tell clinicians how important any one variable was to the outcome (only the importance of the factor to the outcome). Whereas a particular variable may have a strong loading on a factor that is related to outcome, that variable may be only weakly related to outcome. This is because factor analysis groups independent variables based on their relationship to one another, not their relationship to the outcome variable.

For these reasons, factor analysis has a relatively small place in the analysis of medically oriented data. In the behavioral sciences, where we are dealing with constructs that are complicated to measure (e.g., self-esteem, autonomy), the "loss" of single variables is more than compensated for by the strength of the technique for dealing with multiple related independent variables.[12]

6.6 What should I do about missing data on my independent variables?

The problems caused by missing data in bivariate analysis are magnified in multivariable analysis.

Missing data is a problem in all types of analyses. However, the problems caused by missing data in bivariate analysis are magnified in multivariable analysis. Why? Because different subjects will likely have missing values on different variables. Imagine a study of 300 persons with ten independent variables. Each variable has ten missing subjects. In bivariate analysis, the sample size (n) will be 290 persons or 97 percent of your study population. But in multivariable analysis, there will likely be significantly more than ten missing subjects because cases will be dropped from the analysis if they have a missing value on any of the independent variables. At one extreme, if each of the ten variables is missing on a different ten subjects, you will lose ten cases per variable, or 100 cases for ten variables. Your n will be 200 or only 66 percent of your study population. With this amount of missing data, your power to find a significant result is less. Furthermore, your results may not be generalizable to the study population if the missing cases are systematically different from those cases where the data are not missing.

Usually, subjects who have missing values on one variable are more likely to have missing values on other variables. Therefore, the number of cases that

---

[12] For more on factor analysis see: Glantz, S. A. and Slinker, B. K. *Primer of Applied Regression and Analysis of Variance*. New York, NY: McGraw-Hill, 1990, pp. 216–36; Kleinbaum, D. G., Kupper, L. L., and Muller, K. E. *Applied Regression Analysis and Other Multivariable Methods* (2nd edn). Boston, MA: PWS-Kent, 1988, pp. 595–640.

Table 6.4 Methods for dealing with missing data in multivariable analysis.

1. Delete cases with any missing data.
2. Create dichotomous variables to represent missing data.
3. Make additional effort to obtain data.
4. Decrease the number of independent variables in the analysis.
5. Estimate the value of the missing cases.

will need to be dropped will likely be less than 100. How much less depends on how many cases have missing values on more than one independent variable. The opposite extreme from my example would be if all ten variables had missing values for the same ten cases, in which case your multivariable analysis would have no more missing data than your bivariate analysis.

In preparation for deciding how you will deal with missing data in your analysis, it is often helpful to know ahead of time how many missing cases you will have in your multivariable analysis. To determine this, create a variable whose value is 1 if data are missing on any of the independent variables in your analysis and 0 if all the data are present. A simple frequency will then tell you how many cases will be missing in a multivariable analysis that includes all of these variables.

> **TIP**
>
> To determine how many missing cases you will have in your multivariable analysis, create a variable whose value is "1" if the data are missing on any of the independent variables.

After you have determined how much missing data you have, what can you do? Table 6.4 shows five methods for dealing with missing data on independent variables in multivariable analysis. These are discussed in what follows.

Deleting cases with missing values on any independent variable is certainly straightforward and remains the most common method of dealing with missing data in clinical research. However, this strategy has two problems: loss of power and introduction of bias. Although it is easy to determine the loss of power, determining whether you have introduced bias by deleting missing data is more complicated. In general, if the cases are missing at random (such as might occur if different subjects missed answering different questions on a long questionnaire) deleting these cases should not bias the results. In contrast, if the cases with missing data are different from cases without missing data (less compliant with filling out forms, less trusting of interviewers, cognitively impaired, etc.) then deleting them will introduce bias into your results.

To assess whether your data are missing randomly, compare persons with and without missing data on the important independent and dependent variables of your study. If there are no differences, this strengthens the argument that the data are missing randomly, and omitting cases with missing data

TIP

To assess whether your data are missing randomly, compare persons with missing data to persons without missing data on the important independent and dependent variables of your study.

TIP

If you don't exclude the cases with missing values right from the start of the analysis, be sure to tell the reader the sample size for each analysis.

should not bias your study (although there still may be bias owing to unmeasured factors). If there are significant differences between persons with missing data and those without, you can report these differences, so as to better characterize the potential bias in your study. Characterizing how missing cases differ from nonmissing cases is also useful information prior to estimating missing values (method no. 5).

You will note that assessing bias caused by missing cases is similar to assessing bias introduced by subjects choosing not to participate in a study (response bias). Ironically, although the bias introduced by excluding cases with missing data is of equal importance as the bias introduced by nonparticipation, it is much less often reported in published reports. Of course, if you are missing only a few cases, it may not be necessary to evaluate the bias introduced by excluding them.

If you plan on deleting cases in your multivariable analysis that have missing values on any independent variable, you will have to decide how you want to deal with these cases in the univariate and bivariate analyses. You have two choices: You can exclude such cases right from the start of your analysis or you can wait until starting the multivariable analysis.

In published clinical research reports, investigators tend to exclude such cases right from the start. The advantage of this method is that all analyses (univariate, bivariate, and multivariable) in the report then have the same sample size. The disadvantage is that much can be learned from univariate and bivariate analysis. It seems pointless to delete cases from a univariate or bivariate analysis just because they are missing on some other variable that will be part of the multivariable analysis. However, it does make it harder to follow the published analysis if the sample size changes for each analysis.

If the missing data are scattered over a large number of variables it is reasonable to delete cases with missing data on any independent variable. However, if one or two variables account for most of the missing data, it is not worth the loss of a large number of cases on the univariate and bivariate analysis to have the same sample size on all analyses. Remember, if you don't exclude the cases with missing values right from the start of the analysis, you should be careful to tell the reader the sample size for each analysis.

A second strategy for handling missing data is to create multiple dichotomous variables (as you would with a nominal variable or with an interval-independent variable that has a nonlinear relationship with the outcome), with one variable signifying persons with missing data. This strategy was used for dealing with missing data in a study of determinants of kidney transplant failure.[13] The investigators coded the variable – amount of cold ischemia time – as six dichotomous variables: 9–16 hours (yes/no), 17–24 hours (yes/no), 25–36 hours (yes/no), 37–48 hours (yes/no), greater than 48 hours (yes/no), and missing value (yes/no). The reference group was 0–8 hours.

The advantage of using a dichotomous variable to indicate missing data is that it allows all subjects to be included in the multivariable analysis, without making a strong assumption about the missing subjects' values. It has the additional advantage that you get some sense of the bias caused by missing data. In the case of the kidney transplant study, those "yes" on the missing variable had the highest risk of graft failure. This would suggest that those with missing values actually had cold ischemia times greater than the other categories (since long cold ischemia time was associated with higher rates of graft failure). The authors also reported that the fit of models that included a dichotomous variable representing those cases with a missing value on cold ischemia time were not significantly different from the fit of models that excluded cases with missing data.

Since this book is primarily about data analysis, it may surprise you that I have listed "additional effort to obtain data" as the third strategy for dealing with missing data. Won't it be too late to go back to obtain additional data once you are already in the data analysis phase? Certainly, the data collection phase is the most appropriate and efficient time to obtain complete data. I mention this strategy here because the impact of missing data is often felt most acutely in the data analytic phase and sometimes researchers are subsequently able to obtain data that were previously missing. In the case of one study I was involved in, the missing data were in another city. When a thoughtful reviewer pointed out the weakness in our study caused by the missing data, we sent a research assistant on a trip to obtain the data. Some of you may complain that we should have sent a research assistant to collect the data from the other city right from the start. But, research, like any enterprise, is a series of trade-offs between costs (e.g., time, travel) and gains (e.g., more data). It was only after the variable proved to be so important to the analysis (and to the odds that the paper would be published!) that it seemed worth the effort and expense to get the data.

The fourth method for dealing with missing data, decreasing the number of independent variables in the analysis, works only if you have variables that can be eliminated without compromising your analysis. In Section 6.5, I discussed strategies for decreasing the number of independent variables in instances where your sample size is insufficient for the number of variables

> **TIP**
>
> Use of a dichotomous variable to indicate missing data allows all subjects to be included in the multivariable analysis without making a strong assumption about the missing subjects' values.

> **TIP**
>
> Try to eliminate variables with a large number of missing cases.

---

[13] Chertow, G. M., Milford, E. L., Mackenzie, H. S., *et al.* "Antigen-independent determinants of cadaveric kidney transplant failure." *JAMA* **276** (1996): 1732–6.

Table 6.5 Methods of estimating missing values.

Assign the sample mean.
Assign the mean by subgroup (conditional mean).
Model the value of the missing data by using the other covariates in
   the analysis (simple imputation).
Model the value of the missing data by using the other covariates
   in the analysis and include a random component (multiple
   imputation).

in your analysis. These strategies can also help with missing data. There are a few differences worth mentioning. Usually, some variables have more missing data than other variables in the study. Those variables with a large number of missing observations are the variables you should try to eliminate. If you have two related variables and one has a lot more missing data than the other, exclude the one with the greater number of missing observations. For example, education and income are highly correlated. If you have education level for everyone but income level for only 75 percent of the subjects (people are more sensitive about disclosing income than education level), it may be preferable to drop income and use only educational level in the analysis. Since income is not the same as educational level you will certainly lose information by doing this. Only you as the researcher can answer the question of whether you lose more by dropping the cases or by dropping the variable.

The fifth method for dealing with missing data, estimating the value of missing cases, is the most satisfying but also the most dangerous method. It is the most satisfying because you don't lose any cases; it is the most dangerous because you may bias your results in ways that are difficult to predict. Several methods of estimating missing values are shown in Table 6.5.

The simplest method of assigning a missing value for an independent variable is to assign the sample mean (or median) for that variable. (Choose the median if the distribution is skewed.) By assigning the mean/median you are saying that you believe the missing data are occurring randomly and therefore the mean/median provides the best estimate. The benefit of this procedure is that you get to keep the case with missing data in your analysis. However, this method is only sensible if the subjects for whom you are assigning the mean/median have only one or two independent variables with missing values. If, for example, you have 15 cases that have missing values on only one of ten independent variables, by assigning the mean/median for the missing variable you keep all 15 cases in your analysis. They are useful cases because the

> **TIP**
>
> The simplest method of assigning a missing value for an independent variable is to assign the sample mean (or median) for that variable.

information on the other nine independent variables is real. Viewed from the other extreme, if you have 15 cases with missing values on all ten variables, it would serve no purpose to assign them the mean for each of the ten variables. Since all of the data on the independent variables are missing, they contribute no information to your multivariable analysis. Therefore prior to assigning values to missing data make sure that the cases have true values for at least half of the independent variables in your analysis.

When you assign missing values, you may want to assign mean/median values by subgroups rather than using the mean/median for the entire sample. This procedure is referred to as a conditional mean (conditional on the value of other variables). For example, if you have a number of cases with missing data on income, rather than assigning the mean/median for the whole sample, you may assign these cases the mean/median for other subjects of the same educational level and occupational status. Since income is correlated with educational attainment and occupational status, assigning the mean/median by subgroup will likely yield more accurate estimates of missing values.

A more sophisticated method of estimating the mean is to perform a multiple linear or logistic regression analysis using the other independent variables to estimate the missing value. This method, usually referred to as imputation, may allow a more precise estimate of the missing value than assigning the mean/median. For example Smith and colleagues followed 383 patients for 24 months to assess the impact of a primary care intervention on depression.[14] Sixty-two of the subjects had a missing value for income. The researchers therefore used multiple linear regression to estimate the missing values. They included eight independent variables in the model: age, gender, race, education, marital status, employment, physical health rating, and mental health rating. Because all of these variables would be expected to be associated with income (older, white, well-educated, married, employed, healthy men would be expected to have a higher income than younger, nonwhite, less educated, unmarried, unemployed women in poor physical and mental health).

However, as with all the above methods of estimating missing values, if you use the estimated values in your multivariable analysis (as if it were an observed value) you will underestimate the error associated with your coefficients. The reason is that once you have filled in the missing values based on your regression analysis, the computer does not know that the filled-in values have more

> **TIP**
>
> Conditional means will likely yield more accurate estimates of missing values than sample means.

---

[14] Smith, J. L., Rost, K. M., Nutting, P. A., *et al.* "Impact of ongoing primary care intervention on long term outcomes in uninsured and insured patients with depression." *Med. Care* **40** (2002): 1210–22.

"error" than those values that are actually observed. This results in confidence intervals surrounding the estimates that underestimate the actual variability of those estimates.

To overcome this problem, multiple imputation methods allow you to add in a random component.[15] With multiple imputation, you fit a multiple regression or logistic model for the variable with missing values using subjects with complete data on this variable and its important correlates. The fitted model provides an estimate of the mean and variance of each missing value, given the data on the correlates available for that subject. Next, for each missing value, you use a random number generator to simulate an observation from the estimated distribution, under the assumption that interval variables are normally distributed and that dichotomous variables have a binomial distribution. Then the primary analysis is carried out using this data set completed by the imputed missing values. This procedure is repeated at least ten times, and the results are combined using available formulae.[16] Repeating the procedure makes it possible to compute standard errors that take into account the extra uncertainty induced by the imputation, since each data set is completed with different imputed values for the missing data.

Since each method of dealing with missing values has its advantages and disadvantages, some studies will use a combination of methods. For example, Halfon and colleagues conducted a study on access to health services among Latino children.[17] Income was not reported for 13 percent of the sample. They estimated income by replacing missing values with the sample mean. In addition, they created a dichotomous variable representing the cases with missing data on income (in other words, the variable equals 1 if cases are missing and 0 if the cases are not missing). In this way, they were able to provide a value for income for their entire sample and adjust for the possibility that the cases with missing data were different from those without missing data.

One advantage of trying a variety of methods for dealing with missing data (e.g., eliminate cases, assign the mean, impute values) is that you can see if your choice of method makes a difference in the results. It is reassuring to researchers and to readers when different methods of dealing with missing data produce similar findings.

My general guidance on this complicated issue is:

1. Collect your data to minimize missing information.

---

[15] Heitjan, D. F. "What can be done about missing data? Approaches to imputation." *Am. J. Pub. Health* **87** (1997): 548–50.

[16] Rubin, D. B. *Multiple Imputation for Nonresponse in Surveys.* New York, NY: Wiley, 1987.

[17] Halfon, N., Wood, D. L., Valdez, B., *et al.* "Medicaid enrollment and health services access by Latino children in inner-city Los Angeles." *JAMA* **277** (1997): 636–41.

2. Assess how much missing data you have on individual independent variables.

3. If you have one or two independent variables that have significantly more missing cases than your other variables, consider deleting the variables rather than the cases. No matter how important the variable is to your theory, if you have a lot of missing data on that variable, your information is likely to be biased.

4. After you have minimized missing data through steps 1 and 3 above, check to see how many cases have missing values on any of the independent variables you are planning to use in your multivariable model. If you have few cases with missing data, delete them right from the start. It is easier to follow a paper that has the same sample size for all analyses.

5. If you have a large number of cases with missing data, determine if cases with missing values differ from cases without missing values.

6. If missing cases do not differ from nonmissing cases, consider assigning means or conditional means. Before you do this, make sure that the cases have true values for at least half of the independent variables in your analysis. If you have cases that are missing data on most of your independent variables, delete them. With the help of a biostatistician consider using a multiple imputation approach.

7. If missing cases differ from nonmissing cases, you are in a tough spot. Go forward as in step 6, but be clear in your own mind, and to your readers, that assigning values based on the other cases is problematic since you know that the cases with missing values are not the same as nonmissing cases. Of course, excluding them is problematic for the same reason.

8. If possible, try more than one method for dealing with missing data.

9. Read more about the theory and practice of dealing with missing data.[18]

6.7 What should I do about missing data on my outcome variable?

Of those strategies listed in Table 6.4 for dealing with missing data on independent variables, only deleting cases and making additional effort to get the data will work reliably for a missing outcome variable. You can't eliminate your outcome variable (that is, what you are studying). You also cannot

---

[18] Marascuilo, L. A. and Levin, J. R. *Multivariate Statistics in the Social Sciences: A Researcher's Guide*. Monterey, CA: Brooks/Cole Publishing Co., 1983, pp. 64–6; Delucchi, K. L. "Methods for the analysis of binary outcome results in the presence of missing data." *J. Consult. Clin. Psych.* **62** (1994): 569–75; Little, R. J. A. and Rubin, D. B. *Statistical Analysis with Missing Data*. New York, NY: Wiley, 1990; Greenland, S. and Finkle, W. D. "A critical look at methods for handling missing covariates in epidemiologic regression analyses." *Am. J. Epidemiol.* **142** (1995): 1255–64.

estimate your outcome variable prior to the multivariable analysis. The whole purpose of multivariable analysis is to estimate the outcome variable based on the independent variables. For longitudinal studies, data from persons lost to follow-up can contribute to the analysis by censoring observations (Section 3.6). However, it is best not to think of censored observations as missing outcome data. For a censored observation you know what the outcome is at a particular time. You just don't know the outcome beyond that time.

In this section, I want to focus on a strategy for dealing with a missing outcome measure at a particular point in time: multiple imputation. How does multiple imputation work? Remember that multivariable models estimate outcome based on the relationship of the independent variables to the outcome. Once you have estimated outcome based on cases where you have information on independent variables and outcome, you can estimate the outcome of cases where you only have information on the independent variables. What good does this do? By estimating the outcome variable for cases with missing outcomes and including a component that takes into account the variability of this estimate, you can repeat your multivariable analysis with the additional cases and see if your results differ. If they do not, it strengthens the validity of your analysis.

This procedure was used in an evaluation of an HIV-prevention intervention tailored for young gay men.[19] The researchers assessed the sexual risk activities pre- and post-intervention. They found significant decreases in HIV-risk activities between the pre- and post-assessment for the intervention group compared to the non-intervention group. However, of 191 young men who received the pre-intervention assessment, only 103 (54 percent) were available for the post-intervention assessment. This substantial loss of the sample raises questions about the validity of the observed differences.

Even more problematic for the researchers, there were significant differences between those subjects lost to follow-up and those not lost to follow-up. Could these differences, rather than the intervention, explain why there were decreases in sexual risk activities following the intervention? There is no way to definitively answer this question since the subjects were lost and we do not know their ultimate outcome. But we do know something about their pre-intervention behavior.

What the researchers did is to estimate outcome for those subjects who had both pre-intervention and post-intervention interviews using logistic regression analysis. They then used these models to estimate outcome for those cases

[19] Kegeles, S. M., Hays, R. B., and Coates, T. J. "The Mpowerment project: A community-level HIV prevention intervention for young gay men." *Am. J. Pub. Health* **86** (1996): 1129–36.

without a post-intervention assessment. Next, using a multiple imputation procedure, they generated 100 data sets in which the missing outcomes were randomly imputed from the distribution of the missing value according to the logistic model and the observed baseline covariates for the subject. The treatment effect was estimated by the average of the effect estimates for each of the 100 data sets. The standard errors were corrected for the multiple imputation by a factor depending on the variance of the 100 effect estimates. The results of this repeated analysis were similar to those of the analysis in which these cases were excluded. While this strengthened the conclusion of the paper, it certainly does not exclude bias as the explanation of their findings.

Performing the analysis

7.1 What numbers should I assign for dichotomous or ordinal variables in my analysis?

Let's take the simplest case of a dichotomous variable based on an interview question: Do you have a history of diabetes: yes or no?

The equations used to solve multivariable analysis need numerical representations of yes and no. Since this scale only has two points, the numeric distance between the two points can be represented by any two numbers that are separated by one: 0 and 1, 1 and 2, 0 and –1, etc. It doesn't really matter. The sign of the coefficient may change depending on whether you assign "yes" the higher or the lower value, but the coefficient and significance level will be the same (Section 8.3). However, you will not get the same answer if you code your variables such that there is more than one point between the two numbers. For example, coding schemes like +1 and –1 will give you a different answer because there is more than one unit between the two points.

Although any two numbers that are one number apart will give you the same answer, a sensible convention, for both independent and dependent variables, is to use 1 and 0, with 1 representing the presence and 0 representing the absence of the condition. This convention is easy to remember and decreases the chance that you will be confused at the direction of the effect. This coding scheme has another advantage: When a variable is coded this way, the mean of the variable represents the prevalence of the condition. For example, if you have 100 subjects and 10 experience the outcome, the mean of the variable (if coded 0,1) will be $([0 \times 90] + [1 \times 10])/100 = 0.10$. This can be handy when you want to know the prevalence of a risk factor or outcome in a particular group of patients.

For some variables, such as gender, where there is no absence or presence of a condition, assign the 1 to the value that will make the most sense in how you will discuss your results. For example, if your hypothesis is that women

> **TIP**
>
> Code your variables as 1=presence of condition and 0=absence of the condition; then the mean of the variable will be equal to the prevalence of the condition.

Table 7.1 Coding of a dichotomous independent variable and outcome.

Possible coding 1	Possible coding 2
Unemployed = 0; Employed = 1 No treatment = 0; Treatment = 1	Unemployed = 1; Employed = 0 No treatment = 0; Treatment = 1
Possible coding 3	Possible coding 4
Unemployed = 0; Employed = 1 No treatment = 1; Treatment = 0	Unemployed = 1; Employed = 0 No treatment = 1; Treatment = 0

with coronary artery disease receive fewer procedures owing to gender bias, it would be sensible to assign women the 1 and men the 0.

You may feel that I have already belabored the point about coding, but if you are not careful it is so easy to get confused about your results. As you can see from Table 7.1 with just one dichotomous independent variable and one dichotomous outcome there are four possible codings. The different codings will all give you the same result statistically, but the interpretation of the results will be different. For example, if you get confused about how you have coded your variable you may report that a factor increases the risk of an outcome when actually it decreases it. Although this same problem can occur with bivariate analysis, with multiple independent variables it is easier to get confused.

Researchers rarely report in their manuscripts how they have coded their variables. Thus it is unlikely that a miscoded variable will be discovered in peer review. It is up to you to make sure you are reporting your results correctly.

Besides coding your variables in a sensible way and reviewing your work carefully, there are other strategies for minimizing the chance of reporting a result opposite to what your data show. First, name your variables as specifically as you can within the limits of what your statistical packages will allow (usually up to eight characters). For example, it is better to name your variable "femgend" than "gender."

Another useful strategy is to use value labels. The computer will print out the values you have assigned each time you use the variables in the analysis. You are less likely to make a mistake if you see on your printout "1 = employment, 0 = unemployment" next to the variable. Entering value labels takes a bit of extra time at the start of your analysis, but it is worth the effort.

With ordinal variables, the numeric representations of the different levels make no difference so long as the numeric difference between the levels is one unit. So, for example, it would not matter whether a 4-level ordinal variable (very satisfied, satisfied, dissatisfied, very dissatisfied) were coded as 0, 1, 2, 3, or 1, 2, 3, 4 or 9, 10, 11, 12. However, as with dichotomous variables, the direction of the coding will affect the sign of the regression coefficient. So it would matter for the interpretation of the result whether the variable was coded as very satisfied = 1, satisfied = 2, dissatisfied = 3, and very dissatisfied = 4, or very dissatisfied = 1, dissatisfied = 2, satisfied = 3, and very satisfied = 4. As with dichotomous variables the key issue is to keep track of how you have coded your variables and interpret the coefficients accordingly.

7.2 Does it matter what I choose as my reference category for multiple dichotomous ("dummied") variables?

We have reviewed how to create multiple dichotomous variables from a single variable to represent nominal variables (Section 4.2) and how to use multiple dichotomous variables to deal with interval-independent variables that are related to outcome in a nonlinear fashion (Section 4.3.C).

In Section 4.2, I explained that a variable representing the reference group would not be entered into the analysis; rather that the other categories would be compared to this group. Given that, does it matter which category you choose as your reference group? The answer is that your choice of reference group makes a difference in how you report your results and a small difference in the results themselves.

Table 7.2 illustrates the implications of varying your reference group. Assume the data are from a study on the association between ethnicity and access to health care. In column 1, the reference group is white/Caucasian. The odds ratios indicate that African-Americans and Native Americans are a fourth as likely as whites/Caucasians to receive medical care, whereas Latinos, Asian/Pacific Islanders, and other nonwhites are half as likely as whites/Caucasians to receive medical care.

Column 2 lists exactly the same data, but now African-Americans are the reference group. We see that whites are still four times more likely to receive medical care as African-Americans. Latinos, Asian/Pacific Islanders, and other nonwhites are about twice as likely as African-Americans to receive medical care, whereas Native Americans are equally likely as African-Americans to have received medical care.

Although column 1 and 2 are mathematically equivalent, the reporting of the results is slightly different. If the hypothesis of your study was that persons of color have less access to medical care than persons who are white/Caucasian, it would be sensible to have the white/Caucasian group be the reference group as in column 1. This gives you the ability to report to your readers how

Table 7.2 Implications of changing the reference group for dichotomous variables.

	Odds ratio	Odds ratio
White/Caucasian	1.0 (reference)	4.0
African-American	0.25	1.0 (reference)
Latino	0.50	2.0
Asian/Pacific Islander	0.50	2.0
Native American	0.25	1.0
Other nonwhite ethnicity	0.50	2.0

access to medical care differs for persons of color compared to persons who are white/Caucasian. If you made African-Americans your reference group as in column 2, you would not be able to directly compare Latinos, Asian/Pacific Islanders, Native Americans, and other nonwhites to the white/Caucasian group because the reference is to African-Americans. If, however, your research question concerns whether African-Americans are less or more likely to receive medical care than other ethnicities, coding African-Americans as the reference category, as in column 2, is sensible.

For this reason, investigators generally choose the reference category based on the main hypothesis being tested. If you have no main hypothesis, and your dummied variables represent an interval variable (such as age), it is generally easier to report your results in a manner consistent with your empirical findings. For example, if age is associated with increasing (or decreasing) rate of outcome, you should use the extreme category (e.g., the youngest or the oldest subjects) as the reference group. This allows you to summarize your results by saying older persons are more likely (or less likely) than younger persons (the reference category) to experience the outcome. Conversely if the variable underlying the dummied variables has a U-shaped distribution (Section 4.3), it may be best to code the middle group as the reference group so that you can demonstrate the elevated risk at the two extremes.

Which group you choose as your reference group makes a small statistical difference. If you choose the largest group as your reference category, the standard errors will be slightly smaller and the confidence intervals will be somewhat narrower because the model has a larger comparison group and can therefore make more precise estimates. Although this is not a major factor in most studies, if your hypothesis and empirical findings do not lead you to choose a particular category as your reference group, choose the one with the largest sample size.

TIP

If your hypothesis and empirical findings do not lead you to choose a particular category as your reference group, choose the one with the largest sample size.

7.3 How do I enter interaction terms into my analysis?

In Section 1.4, I explained that an interaction occurs when the association of an independent variable on outcome is changed by the value of a third variable. How do you deal with interaction terms in a multivariable analysis?

> The most common method of incorporating an interaction in a multivariable model is to create a product term.

The most common method of incorporating an interaction in a multivariable model is to create a product term. This is done by creating a variable whose value is the product of two independent variables (i.e., the two variables multiplied by each other). A product term between two independent variables is referred to as a two-way interaction or a primary interaction. A product term between three independent variables is referred to as a three-way interaction or a secondary interaction.

In Section 1.4, I reviewed an example of an interaction between gender and ST elevations. The coding for the product term for male gender and ST elevations is shown in Table 7.3. Note that the two variables male gender (yes/no) and ST elevations (yes/no) divide the sample into four groups: men with ST elevations, men without ST elevations, women with ST elevations, and women without ST elevations. Each cell has its own unique combination of these two variables. In bold is the value of the product term. Note how the product term highlights those subjects who have both risk factors (male and ST elevations).

To determine if an interaction was present between male gender and ST elevations, the authors entered the product term into their multiple logistic regression analysis, along with the two variables constituting the product term (male gender and ST elevations). If there had been no interaction, meaning the effect of the two risk factors on outcome (heart attack) is captured by the two variables, male gender and ST elevations, then the product term would have been nonsignificant. The authors would have established that there was no interaction between male gender and ST elevations. Instead the product term was significant, indicating that there was an interaction. In this case the sign on the product term was negative, indicating that the effect of being male and having ST elevations had significantly less impact on the likelihood of heart attack than you would have expected from the individual effects of male gender and hypertension.

Because a product term describes the relationship between two risk factors and an outcome, it can only be interpreted as an interaction if the two risk factors (in this case male gender and ST elevations) are in the model. If you enter only the product term, without assessing the individual risk factors in the model and the product term is significant, you don't know if the product is significant because there is an interaction between the risk factors or because the risk of outcome is significantly higher when both risk factors are present

Table 7.3 Creation of an interaction (product) term.

Male gender	ST elevations	
	Yes (= 1)	No (= 0)
Yes (= 1)	$1 \times 1 = \mathbf{1}$	$1 \times 0 = \mathbf{0}$
No (= 0)	$0 \times 1 = \mathbf{0}$	$0 \times 0 = \mathbf{0}$

Because a product term describes the relationship between two risk factors and an outcome, it can only be interpreted as an interaction if the two risk factors are in the model.

(compared to subjects who do not have both risk factors). In this example, if the investigators did not include the separate variables for male gender and ST elevations, and entered only the product term, the product term certainly would have been statistically significant and positive (since males with ST elevations are at higher risk of heart attack than the rest of the sample). But the importance of the product term is that it is statistically significant and negative when both male gender and ST elevations are in the model.

Although I have stressed the importance of initially including the variables that constitute the product term in the model, it would not be incorrect to have a model that had only the product term. If, for example, the two variables constituting the product term are not on their own statistically associated with the outcome in initial models, it would be acceptable to drop them from subsequent models.

An alternative method for incorporating product terms into your analysis is to create multiple dichotomous variables representing the interaction. Look back at Table 7.3. There are four distinct codings of the variables gender and ST elevations. Rather than entering three variables representing gender, ST elevations, and the product of gender and ST elevations, you could create three dichotomous variables:

men with ST elevations (yes/no)
men without ST elevations (yes/no)
women with ST elevations (yes/no)

The reference group would be women without ST elevations. One advantage of this coding is that it will be easier for you to see and interpret the impact of the combinations of gender and ST elevations on outcome. A second advantage is that you can see the effect of the double-exposed group (male and ST elevations) compared to persons with only one risk factor and persons with neither risk factor (the reference group). (When you use product terms you see the risk of the doubly-exposed persons compared to persons with only one or no risk factors.)

A disadvantage of multiple dichotomous variable coding is that if you are looking at multiple interactions involving a particular variable (e.g., male gender) you will have to create more additional variables than you would if you were using product terms. For example, if in addition to the interaction between male gender and ST elevation you wanted to describe the interaction between gender and congestive heart failure you would need three variables: men with congestive heart failure, men without congestive heart failure, and women with congestive heart failure. If you wanted instead to create an interaction term you would enter only two variables: (1) congestive heart failure and (2) the product of congestive heart failure and male gender. You would not have to add a variable for male gender because it is already in the model.

7.4 How do I enter time into my proportional hazards or other survival analysis?

For linear and logistic regression you need only enter your independent and dependent variables. For proportional hazards analysis and other types of survival analysis you must also enter a time for each subject. The time is the interval from a subject's participation in the study to the date the subject experienced an outcome, was lost to follow-up, was withdrawn, or completed the study.

The starting point ("zero time") will depend on the kind of study you are performing, as shown in Table 7.4. For a randomized controlled trial the starting time is the date of randomization. For a trial that prospectively enrolls subjects but does not randomize them to a treatment, the starting point is usually the date of enrollment.

In observational studies, the choice of starting point is complicated. The goal is to choose a starting point that best represents the start of the process you are studying. For example, in evaluating the rate of death in patients with coronary artery disease, the starting point should be the onset of coronary artery disease. But how do you determine the date that coronary artery disease began? Is the starting point the date that the patient first developed chest pain? This sounds good, but remember some patients have coronary artery disease without ever having chest pain. Others have chest pain for years from some other cause before they develop coronary artery disease. Also, some patients will not remember their first episode of chest pain; they may report that they have had chest pain for "years."

What can you do to get a more precise starting time? You could use the date coronary angiography first demonstrated coronary artery stenosis. This starting date has the advantage of being the most objective (angiography is the gold standard for diagnosing coronary artery disease). But many patients never

Table 7.4 Starting time for survival analysis.

Type of study	Start time
Randomized controlled trial	Date of randomization
Nonrandomized trial	Enrollment into trial
Observational study	Varies:
	Date of first visit
	Date of first symptom
	Date of diagnosis
	Date of start of treatment

require angiography, and access to care and patients' willingness to undergo testing will affect whether and when they have angiography.

Often with observational studies, no one starting point truly represents the onset of the disease process for all participants. You have to choose the best one you have available. In a study of patients seen in a clinical setting this may be the date the patient first presented for medical care. In a prospective cohort study the starting point may be the first cohort visit. Although not ideal, date of first visit has been used in many studies. Notably, many natural-history studies of HIV infection use the date of first visit because this was the first date that the participant was documented to be HIV-antibody positive. The actual disease process had begun months to years earlier when the person actually seroconverted to HIV. Although use of first visit did bias the results from these cohorts and has led to some inaccurate observations, these studies were nonetheless extremely helpful in understanding the nature of HIV disease.[1]

In conclusion, choose the starting point that best represents the start of the process you are studying and clearly state the choice in the methods section of your paper.

The endpoint for survival analysis is the date of the outcome of interest or the censor date (Section 3.6). For subjects lost to follow-up prior to outcome the censor date is the last date of known follow-up. For subjects who did not experience an outcome and were not lost to follow-up, the censor date is the end date of the study (assuming intention-to-treat analysis for patients who are withdrawn).

In some studies there may be ambiguity about the appropriate censor date because the investigators have access to supplemental sources of data about study participants. Analysis of survival time following an AIDS diagnosis

[1] For a perspective on the biases of prevalent cohorts of HIV-infected persons see: Alcabes, P., Pezzotti, P., Phillips, A. N., *et al.* "Long-term perspective on the prevalent-cohort biases in studies of human immunodeficiency virus progression." *Am. J. Epidemiol.* **146** (1997): 543–51.

provides a good illustration of this principle. Let's say you want to determine whether persons who are lost to follow-up in your study have died. You know that death certificates are part of the public record and it is therefore possible to determine whether subjects who are lost to follow-up have died. However, you are also aware that there is usually a delay between when a subject dies and when you will learn about their death from a local, state, or national death registry. Conversely, matching with a death registry may enable you to learn about the deaths of some participants sooner than you otherwise would have. This can occur if you interview subjects only periodically (e.g., every six months to a year) but perform frequent reviews with a death registry (e.g., weekly to monthly). How should you deal with this supplementary information about survival?

In San Francisco, we follow all persons who are diagnosed with AIDS by reviewing their medical records every six months. We also review all of the death certificates in San Francisco weekly. Each year we perform a match with the National Death Index.[2] This index covers the deaths of all persons in the United States. Thus, when someone dies we almost certainly find out about it. We need to decide what is the appropriate date to use as the last date of follow-up for someone who is not known to have died. The algorithm we use to determine this date is somewhat complicated but illustrates the types of decisions you must make about the last date of follow-up.

For subjects not known to have died, we check the medical record for the date of the last medical visit or laboratory test. What about people whose records show no recent entries and yet are not listed as being dead? These people either died outside San Francisco (because if they died in San Francisco we would know it since we do weekly reviews of San Francisco's death certificates), moved, switched their site of care, or stopped receiving medical care altogether. What should our last date of follow-up be for these individuals?

For persons not known to have died, with no recent medical follow-up, we use for their censor date the date to which the National Death Index is current at the time we match our database with theirs. The National Death Index receives all state death certificates and updates their computer files for the deaths that occurred in a calendar year within 12 months of the end of the calendar year. For example, if we performed our match in June of 2005, the data would be complete for the calendar year of 2003. For those cases lost to follow-up, we would use December 31, 2003 as the censor date.

---

[2] For information about the National Death Index (for the United States) along with an application for matching your data with the Index see: www.cdc.gov.nchs/r&d/ndi/ndi.htm.

Of course, matches with the National Death Index are not perfect. The index is not 100 percent complete (nothing ever is). Also, it is possible that a case is listed in the National Death Index but we are unable to match with it because we have incorrect identifying information (e.g., the wrong date of birth). A more conservative strategy than using the date for which the National Death Index is current would be to use the last dates listed in the medical records of those patients not known to have died. The problem with this strategy is that it underestimates survival because it counts those deaths that we know occurred after the last date of follow-up, but not the survival time beyond the date of follow-up. At the other extreme, we could censor everyone at the date of analysis. Supporting this strategy is the fact that most San Francisco AIDS patients die in San Francisco and we review the death certificates weekly. Therefore, in most cases we will know promptly if someone has died. However, using the date of analysis would overestimate survival because it would count all of the follow-up time but would miss some of the deaths. Our method is something of a compromise.

As you can see, the date of censor can be quite a complicated issue. Your choice will affect the survival time. van Benthem and colleagues illustrate this using a similar example to mine, that of AIDS incubation time (time from HIV seroconversion to AIDS diagnosis).[3] In their example, they show that AIDS incubation time varies based on when participants are censored. When participants with no known AIDS diagnoses are censored at the date of their last visit, incubation time is underestimated (because information about deaths from registry-matches is included but additional AIDS-free time is not included). When participants with no known AIDS diagnoses are censored at the date of analysis, incubation time is overestimated (because it assumes that the information from the registries is complete, which it is not). In their example, they advocate for an alternative method: Persons seen in the year prior to the analysis, who are not in the AIDS registry, are censored at the date of analysis; persons not seen in the year prior to the date of analysis and persons who developed AIDS more than a year after their last visit are censored one year after their last visit.

> **TIP**
>
> Choose a censor date that balances information about outcomes with information about outcome-free time.

The most interesting thing about the analysis of van Benthem and colleagues is that they demonstrate that differences in AIDS incubation time reported by different studies may actually be caused by differences in the censoring techniques. Thus, in handling supplementary information, I recommend you balance information about outcomes with information about outcome-free time

---

[3] van Benthem, B.H.B., Veugelers, P.J., Schecter, M.T., *et al.* "Modelling the AIDS incubation time: Evaluation of three right censoring strategies." *AIDS* **11** (1997): 834–5.

Table 7.5 Illustration of time calculations for individual subjects.

Subject	Start Date	Did heart attack occur?	Date of heart attack	Date of last follow-up	Time (days)
1	May 1, 2004	Yes	May 1, 2005	August 1, 2005	365
2	May 1, 2004	No	Not applicable	August 1, 2005	457
3	August 1, 2004	No	Not applicable	August 1, 2005	365
4	May 1, 2004	No	Not applicable	July 1, 2004	61

and try to be consistent with how others in your field have dealt with this issue.

Once you have settled on the start date and end date for each subject, the difference between these dates represents the survival time for each subject in your analysis.

Table 7.5 illustrates calculations of time for different types of subjects. Subjects were enrolled between May 1, 2004 and August 1, 2004 and were followed until August 1, 2005 unless they dropped out or were withdrawn. The outcome of interest is heart attack.

Subject 1 experienced a heart attack one year (365 days) after enrollment but continued to be followed after the outcome. This is common in clinical studies. You might follow someone beyond their main outcome of interest because you are assessing the development of side effects or a secondary outcome (e.g., death). However, note that to determine time to heart attack for this analysis, you subtract the start date from the date of outcome, not the date of last follow-up. Let's contrast this with subject 2. This subject did not have a heart attack. Therefore time is the difference between the start date and the date of last follow-up. Subject 3, like subject 2, did not experience a heart attack. But this subject enrolled in the study later than subjects 1 and 2. Therefore, even though the subject stayed till the end of the study, the subject would be censored at 365 days. Subject 4 dropped out of the study and is censored at 61 days.

The four subjects shown in Table 7.5 illustrate two important points about survival analysis.

- Survival analysis tracks length of time without reference to calendar time. If you changed the decade in which the study occurred by subtracting ten years from all the dates, you would get the same survival time. This is the reason that many analyses adjust for year of diagnosis or birth cohort (i.e., year or period of years of birth).
- There is no special designation for cases that are censored. All subjects that do not experience an outcome are censored. The only difference between

subjects 2, 3, and 4, from the computer's point of view, is the amount of time they contribute to the analysis.

There is another method for incorporating time into a proportional hazards model: Use of age of subject rather than study time. Using age instead of study time makes sense in observational studies of healthy persons. This is because the hazard of an outcome such as death for a 55-year-old man observed for 15 years is likely to be more similar to the hazard for a 55-year-old man observed for 5 years, than that for a 40-year-old man observed for 15 years.

Korn and colleagues argue persuasively for the use of age instead of study time for observational studies of healthy persons drawn from national surveys.[4] However, their empirical analysis demonstrates that the more usual method of study time, with adjustment for subject's age, produces unbiased estimates even when age may be a more appropriate time scale.

Although the use of age in place of study time has its adherents, it is not commonly done, even for surveys of healthy persons. It would certainly not be appropriate in studies of persons with disease. In persons with an illness (e.g., cancer, heart disease) the amount of time that they have the disease is likely to be more closely related to their rate of outcome (e.g., death) than their age.

If you do choose to use age as your time scale, it is important to adjust for birth cohort. Otherwise, your model will not take into account treatment changes that have occurred during the lives of your participants.

7.5 What about subjects who experience their outcome on their start date?

It sometimes happens that subjects experience their outcome on their start date. If this occurs, the time for such subjects would be zero. Since, at time zero, by definition, none of the subjects have experienced an outcome, persons with time equal to zero must be excluded from the analysis. Is this fair? Can you do anything to prevent this?

To answer this question, you have to distinguish those cases where the outcome truly occurred on the start date from those cases where the start date and the outcome are *recorded* as occurring on the same date, but the start date is really unknown. I will illustrate with a few examples.

Imagine you are studying hospital survival with a rapidly progressive disease, such as adult respiratory distress syndrome (ARDS). A certain number of patients will die on their day of admission to the hospital. In this case, if you

---

[4] Korn, E. L., Graubard, B. I., and Midthune, D. "Time-to-event analysis of longitudinal follow-up of a survey: Choice of the time scale." *Am. J. Epidemiol.* **145** (1997): 72–80.

TIP

The use of a day as the unit of survival analysis is arbitrary. Hours may be a more appropriate unit for rapidly progressive diseases.

computed survival in days, patients who died on their date of admission would appear to have a survival of zero days and would be excluded from the analysis. Clearly, this is not what you would want. The true survival time for these patients is in hours. Our use of a day as the unit of survival analysis is arbitrary. For this example, you should switch your unit of analysis to hours. This will work well for ARDS or other diseases that have a very rapid progression time. Day is the convention for most survival analyses because improvement and worsening of most clinical conditions occur in days not in hours.

Consider a more complex example: How to categorize patients who are diagnosed with AIDS and die on the same day. If you were to review data from the San Francisco Health Department's AIDS registry, you would discover that some of our cases have the same date for AIDS diagnosis and death. There are two reasons for this. In some cases, HIV-infected patients without an AIDS diagnosis are admitted to the hospital, diagnosed with an AIDS-defining illness for the first time, and die the same day they are admitted. In this case, as with the ARDS example, there is a real survival time, measured in hours. Unfortunately, our records do not contain the hour of AIDS diagnosis or death. In other cases, the patients' date of diagnosis is the same as their date of death because they are diagnosed by the medical examiner (coroner). In these cases, it is unclear what the true survival time is because you don't know if they had an AIDS illness for a short or a long time before death. How do we deal with these two types of cases, both of whom have a survival time of zero?

For cases diagnosed on the day of admission, we consider their survival to be 0.5 days. The half-day acknowledges that the death truly occurred after the diagnosis of AIDS, but after an interval of less than one day. (Some statistical software programs will automatically add 0.5 units to cases with a survival time of zero. However, you as the investigator should determine whether this is a reasonable assumption or not.) For those cases diagnosed by the medical examiner, we exclude the case because we do not know what the true interval is between diagnosis and death.

The AIDS registry of the New York City Health Department has an even more complicated problem. Unlike San Francisco, they only record the month and year of AIDS diagnosis. Thus a case who died in the same calendar month as their AIDS diagnosis would have a survival time of zero. They therefore have a large proportion of cases (11 percent) with a survival time of zero.[5]

How do the investigators deal with New York City AIDS cases with survival time equal to zero? They exclude them from the analysis. This may be

---

[5] Blum, S., Singh, T. P., Gibbons, J., *et al*. "Trends in survival among persons with acquired immunodeficiency syndrome in New York City." *Am. J. Epidemiol.* **139** (1994): 351–61.

problematic. To the extent that such persons truly had a short survival, the investigators' method will artificially lengthen survival by excluding these subjects. Because such cases represented a large group, the investigators assessed whether the survivors were different from other participants. In fact they were: They were more likely to be female, persons of color, and injection drug users. This illustrates another important point. You cannot always eliminate bias whether caused by loss of cases or some other reason. Nonetheless, you should always investigate it and describe it to your readers (as these authors did).

7.6 What about subjects who have a survival time shorter than physiologically possible?

It sometimes happens that subjects experience their outcome so soon after their start date that the survival time is not physiologically possible. This is most likely to pose a dilemma with slowly progressive diseases, for which the physiology of the disease does not support a survival time of a day or a week. For example, what do you do with a subject enrolled in a study of cancer incidence who is diagnosed with lung cancer a week after enrollment? We know it takes years from the first malignant cell division to the time that the cancer is detectable. Do you exclude the subject who is diagnosed with cancer a week after enrollment? If you say yes, what about the subject diagnosed a month after, or a year after? The longer the time, the murkier the decision.

As with most things, prevention is the best defense. To avoid this problem, develop rigorous pre-enrollment criteria to ensure that subjects do not have the outcome at the time the study starts (at least as best as can be determined). Staying with the example of lung cancer, you may want subjects to have a respiratory symptom review and a pre-enrollment chest x-ray.

Unfortunately, certain diseases are difficult to rule out without subjecting participants to very invasive tests (which would increase the expense of your trial and decrease enrollment). For example, some HIV-infected patients have *Pneumocystis carinii* pneumonia (PCP) with minimal or no symptoms and normal chest x-rays. If you wanted to be sure that subjects do not have PCP prior to enrolling them in a PCP-prevention trial, you would have to perform bronchoscopy on all of them. However, it is not feasible or ethical to subject asymptomatic persons to an invasive test prior to enrollment in a trial to prevent the disease. Instead, most investigators performing studies on preventing PCP limit the pre-enrollment evaluation to a chest x-ray and symptom review. Invariably, a few patients are diagnosed with PCP just days after enrollment.

> **TIP**
>
> Develop rigorous pre-enrollment criteria to ensure that subjects do not have the outcome at the time the study starts.

Besides being difficult to diagnose, PCP usually develops slowly, over a period of weeks. If a patient is diagnosed with PCP a week after starting a treatment protocol designed to prevent PCP, should the patient be considered a treatment failure (since the outcome of interest occurred while the patient was on the study) or should the subject be deleted from the analysis (since the subject almost certainly had PCP at the time of enrollment)? This is a judgment call. What most investigators do is to exclude those cases of PCP that occur within twenty-eight days of enrollment.[6] Cases that occur after twenty-eight days are considered treatment failures.

In considering this example you may wonder: Would it not be safer to include people who develop PCP after enrollment in the study no matter how soon after the start date? In support of this, remember that in a randomized controlled trial implausibly early outcomes should be evenly distributed in the different arms of the study. Therefore, including these early-outcome subjects will not bias your analysis, although it will result in your reporting higher treatment failure rates in the different arms of the study. But, in observational studies, improbably early outcomes would not necessarily be evenly distributed in the different arms of your study and could thus be a source of bias in your study.

> **TIP**
>
> Even if you have a-priori criteria for exclusion it is best to have the decision to exclude a subject made by a review committee that is blind to the treatment assignment.

My general advice in this area is develop pre-enrollment criteria that will lower the chance of implausibly early outcomes. Beyond this, decide ahead of time what you will do if a subject develops the outcome of interest a day after your study begins. If it will be important to you to exclude such early outcomes, develop objective exclusion criteria for subjects prior to the start of a study. Even if you have a-priori criteria for exclusion it is best to have a review committee that is blind to the treatment assignment make the decision to exclude a subject.

At times, it may be worth excluding early outcomes as a way of testing a hypothesis on the cause-and-effect relationship between your risk factor and outcome. For example, in the study of cholesterol level and mortality discussed in Section 4.3.A, the investigators excluded cancers that occurred in the first four years of the study. They did this to test whether low cholesterol levels might be a consequence of cancer that was present but unsuspected at the time of entry into the cohort. When they excluded these cases, the relationship between low cholesterol level and cancer persisted, suggesting that the relationship between the low cholesterol level and mortality was not a consequence of unsuspected cancer at the time of enrollment.

---

[6] Leung, G. S., Feigal, D. W., Montgomery, A. B., *et al.* "Aerosolized pentamadine for prophylaxis against *pneumocystis carinii* pneumonia." *N. Engl. J. Med.* **323** (1990): 769–75; Golden, J. A., Katz, M. H., Chernoff, D. N., *et al.* "A randomized comparison of once-monthly or twice-monthly high-dose aerosolized pentamadine prophylaxis." *Chest* **104** (1993): 743–50.

7.7 How do I incorporate time into my Poisson analysis?

You will remember from Section 3.11, that Poisson regression (or the related procedure of negative binomial regression) can be used to compare the incidence rates of two or more groups with statistical adjustment for other variables.

An incidence rate is the number of (first-time) events in a group divided by the total at-risk time of the group. The at-risk time for most medical studies is person-years. To determine the total at-risk time for the group, you need to sum the amount of at-risk time each participant contributes to the analysis. The process of calculating the at-risk time for each participant is very similar to the process of determining time for survival analysis. Each person has a zero time (start time) and is at risk until they either experience the outcome (counted in the numerator), develops an outcome that precludes development of the outcome under study, is withdrawn, or is no longer being followed.

The assumptions underlying calculation of incidence rates are similar to those underlying survival analysis such as proportional hazards analysis. Specifically, for incidence rates to be valid the likelihood of outcome for subjects that drop out, develop an alternative outcome, or are withdrawn, must be the same as that for subjects who continue in the study. There must also be no temporal changes during the period being summarized by a single rate.

An important difference in the calculation of total at-risk time between survival analysis and incidence rates is that it is possible to calculate a total at-risk time for a population without having the risk time for individuals. To illustrate, look back at the study on whether pregnancy increases the risk of stroke (Section 3.11). Since there was not a cohort study into which subjects were enrolled, the investigators did not know when women in the catchment area became pregnant. This is essential information for calculating individual at-risk time. Nonetheless, it was still possible to estimate the group time at-risk. To do so, the investigators first determined the person-time "at risk during pregnancy" based on the average number of spontaneous and induced abortions, still births, and live births in the population and the average length of each pregnancy state. The person-time not at risk owing to pregnancy was calculated by subtracting the estimate of person-time spent pregnant from the total time at risk. To calculate the total time at risk the investigators simply needed to know the population of girls and women aged 15 to 44 years (the study inclusion criteria) in their catchment area, a number that would be available in any locality through census data. This number of girls and women could then be multiplied by the years that strokes were ascertained (1988–1991) to determine the total time at risk. Although calculating group at-risk time based on population registries and estimates of lengths of time spent in different pregnancy states is certainly less precise than summing individual at-risk times from a cohort of women of reproductive age, the latter would have been unfeasible given the low rates of stroke in pregnant women.

7.8 What are variable selection techniques?

Variable selection techniques are automatic procedures that determine which independent variables will be included in a multivariable model. They can also determine the order in which the variables enter the model. The parameters of the algorithms are determined by the investigator.

I have already referred to variable selection techniques as a flawed strategy for decreasing the number of independent variables in your analysis. This may be necessary because of an insufficient sample size for the number of independent variables in your model (Section 6.5). The other major reason for using selection procedures is that you want to determine the minimum number of independent variables necessary to accurately estimate outcome. This is particularly important in the development of diagnostic and prognostic models (Sections 2.4 and 2.5, respectively) because the fewer the variables the more likely clinicians are to remember and use them.

In Section 2.4, I detailed a decision rule for determining which patients presenting with chest pain to an emergency room were probably having acute ischemia. The investigators used forward stepwise-regression to create the prediction rule. Using forward selection they evaluated a total of fifty-nine clinical characteristics; the selection algorithm chose the seven variables that best accounted for ischemia. If instead the investigators developed a model using all fifty-nine characteristics, it would undoubtedly have had better diagnostic capability than the seven-variable model. But what clinician would use a fifty-nine variable model in a clinical setting? Patients would require hospital admission just so that their physician would have enough time to record the values of the fifty-nine clinical characteristics and compute each patient's probability of ischemia!

Most statistical software packages offer a variety of variable selection techniques (Table 7.6). What all selection methods have in common is that they use statistical criteria to decide which variables should enter the model and the order of the variables entering the model.

Using forward selection, the model will select the variable most strongly related to the outcome and enter it first into the model. In fact, you can predict which variable will enter first in a forward-selection model by looking at your bivariate analysis. The variable with the strongest association with your outcome in the bivariate analysis will enter first. You will not be able to

Table 7.6 Methods of variable selection.

Type of selection technique	Method	Advantages and disadvantages
Forward	Enters variables into the model sequentially. The order is determined by the variable's association with outcome (variables with strongest association enter first) after adjustment for any variables already in the model.	Best suited for dealing with studies where the sample size is small. Does not deal well with suppresser effects.
Backward	Deletes variables from the model sequentially. The order is determined by the variable's association with outcome (variables with weakest association leave first) after adjustment for any variables already in the model.	Better for assessing suppresser effects than forward selection.
Best subset	Determines the subset of variables that maximizes a specified measure.	Computationally difficult.
None (all variables)	Enters all variables at the same time.	Including all variables may be problematic if there are many independent variables and you have a small sample size.

predict the second variable that will enter simply by looking at the bivariate analysis because the model will choose the variable that best improves the fit of the model after adjusting for the first variable. This may not be the variable with the second strongest association with outcome in the bivariate analysis. It depends how closely these two independent variables are related to each other. If they are very closely related, it is possible that once you know the value of the first variable, the value of the second variable does not substantially improve the fit of your model. Instead a variable that is less strongly associated with outcome in the bivariate analysis, but unrelated to the first variable that entered, may be the second strongest variable in improving the fit of your model.

Forward selection will continue to evaluate each variable for how it improves the fit of your model. When none of the remaining variables significantly improves the fit, it will stop entering variables. You as the researcher must decide what statistical cut-off to use for determining that the addition of another variable does not significantly improve the fit of the model. With lower cut-offs fewer variables will be included, but you will be more likely to miss important confounders. With higher cut-offs you will be less likely to miss important confounders but you will have a model with more variables in it.

Forward models can be modified to allow you to delete variables that were significant on entry into the model but are not statistically significant after other variables have entered. To do this, you will need to specify a statistical cut-off for removal of a variable that was already entered. You may want to set a less stringent (higher P value) cut-off to remove a variable once entered, or use the same cut-off for both. Forward-selection models with deletion of entered variables that are no longer significant will produce a model with potentially fewer variables than simple forward selection.

Backward selection is similar to forward selection – except it proceeds backwards! At step one all variables enter into the model. If you have ten independent variables, all ten will enter in this step, no matter how unrelated they are to outcome. The algorithm then assesses which of the ten variables in the model is least important in accounting for the outcome, and deletes it, so that there are now nine variables in the model. The model then assesses which of the nine is least important in accounting for the outcome. It deletes this variable and then repeats the process until all the remaining variables are significantly associated with the outcome. At this point no further variables are deleted. As with forward selection, the researcher determines what statistical cut-off will be used for retaining (or not deleting) a variable.

You may, at first, think that forward or backward selection would arrive in the same place just by different routes, like two cars converging on a city from opposite directions. While it is a sign of a robust model when forward and backward selection give you the same answer, this does not always occur. The reason that forward and backward selection do not necessarily produce the same answer is that the importance of a particular variable often depends on what other variables are in the model at the time of selection. A variable may be statistically important when a variable (or a group of variables) is in the model and yet not significant when that variable (or group of variables) is not in the model. This is referred to as a suppresser effect (Section 1.3). In forward selection, it is less likely that the variable needed to demonstrate the suppresser effect would be in the model. For this reason, backward selection is more likely to detect a variable that is significant only when the suppresser variable is in the model.

Forward selection is preferable over backward selection when your sample size is small for the number of independent variables in your analysis or when you have concerns about multicollinearity. This is because in backward selection all the variables are in the model initially. If you have doubts about the

TIP

Backward selection is more likely to demonstrate a suppresser effect than forward selection.

TIP

Forward selection is preferable to backward selection when your sample size is small for the number of independent variables in your analysis or when you have concerns about multicollinearity.

reliability of a model with all the variables in it, then there is reason to worry about having this model be the starting point for decisions on which variables to delete.

In best subset regression, the computer chooses the best combination of variables from all possible models. In the case of an analysis with only five variables, there are thirty-one possible combinations of variables (including models that have one, two, three, four, and five variables). The number of possible combinations increases exponentially as you increase the number of possible variables. "Best" is determined by a specified measure of the ability of the model to account for the outcome. For example, in multiple linear regression, you could have the computer choose the combination of variables that produces the highest adjusted R^2 (Section 8.2.A).

In some ways, best subset regression is hard to argue with. It is, after all, the best statistical answer to the question. However, because of the computational time involved, this technique cannot always be done. For logistic regression and proportional hazards analysis, best subset regression is usually modified to include the best possible combination of two variables, then of three variables, then of four variables, up to the maximum number of variables in your model (some programs will limit the maximum number of variables to ten). This is a simplification in that the computer is not comparing models of different size to one another (e.g., comparing those that have five variables to those that have four variables). Also, just because it is the best statistical answer does not mean it truly reflects the physiology of what you are studying. Confounders may be included in the model while the main effects are missing. Conversely, confounders that may change the coefficients of certain variables in important ways may be omitted.

Although I have described these selection algorithms as distinct, there are many hybrids. A popular hybrid is to enter certain variables in the model at the start of the analysis and not allow them to be deleted even if they are not significantly related to the outcome. The computer then enters the remaining independent variables in a forward or backward manner. This strategy works well when there are certain variables that you absolutely want in your analysis for theoretical or practical reasons. For example, if every prior analysis of your outcome shows that age is an important confounder, it makes sense to add age right at the start, and not allow it to leave the model.

Forward- and backward-selection techniques can be modified to minimize the effect of missing data in your analysis. With forward or backward selection, after you have derived your model, you can rerun it with only the variables that entered (or were not deleted). By rerunning the model with a smaller number of variables, missing data on the excluded variables will no longer result in missing cases in the multivariable model. With backward selection, you can rerun the model with each deletion of a variable, so that each iteration of the model has a larger sample size. With both forward- and backward-selection techniques you will need to specify what level of statistical significance should result in the inclusion or exclusion of a variable. Most researchers use a P value of < 0.05 or, for smaller sample sizes, a P value of <0.10 or <0.15. However, just because a variable does not meet the P value criterion does not mean that it is unimportant. The algorithm does not evaluate whether entry of the variable changes the coefficients of the other variables in the model. While it is unlikely that a variable that has no association with outcome will make a significant impact on the other coefficients, it is possible that a variable that is marginally associated with the outcome will change the coefficients of the other independent variables in important ways. This is one reason many researchers favor higher (less restrictive) cut-offs than $P < 0.05$.

TIP

Don't use selection algorithms!

Now that you understand the different types of selection algorithms, I have one more piece of advice: If at all possible DON'T USE THEM! With all of the variable selection procedures you run the risk of the model eliminating (or not selecting) a variable that is on the causal pathway to your outcome, in favor of a variable that is a confounder. Because forward and backward selection algorithms evaluate variables singly, there is a possibility that your final model will not include two variables that together are important in changing your main effect. Also, a variable may be very important in explaining an outcome, and yet get kicked out of the model because it is related to a variable that is already in the model.

Therefore, you (not some computer algorithm) should determine, based on your theoretical understanding and your empirical findings, what variables to include in your model. Without a variable selection algorithm, all variables that you specify will be entered simultaneously (this is sometimes referred to as forcing all variables into the model). You will not have to worry about the possibility of missing suppresser effects or important changes in coefficients caused by exclusion of a modest confounder. Another advantage of all variable models is that when you submit your paper for publication, you will not have to explain why certain variables are not included in your model. While one can certainly defend exclusion of a variable in selection models because it was not statistically related to the outcome, the reviewer may cite the possibility that the missing variable is a modest confounder or a suppresser variable. With all your variables entered into your model you can demonstrate that the variable of interest is included and does or does not affect the outcome and the relationship of the other independent variables to the outcome.

As with other rules of thumb, there is an exception. It's okay to use a selection algorithm if your goal is to identify the best possible diagnostic model with the fewest number of variables. With predictive models for diagnosis and prognosis (Sections 2.4 and 2.5, respectively) we are not concerned with causality. If knowing the value of a risk factor enables you to diagnose accurately a condition it does not matter whether the variable is or is not causally associated with the condition. Also, diagnostic models are much more likely to be used by busy clinicians if they have a small number of variables.

7.9 My model won't converge. What should I do?

You may sometimes get a message that your logistic or proportional hazards or Poisson model won't converge. What this means is that the computer cannot solve the equation. There are several reasons this can happen. In the simplest cases, you have made an error in your coding. If you have coded an outcome variable, such that everyone has the same outcome (this can happen if you are not careful with your if/then statements), the computer cannot solve the equation. It cannot compute the odds of outcome versus no outcome if everyone has the outcome.

> **TIP**
>
> Models will not converge if you have defined a subgroup in which no (or very few) outcomes have occurred.

Recognizing this, you can probably imagine another reason that a model will not converge: You have too few outcomes for the number of independent variables in your model (Section 6.4). Your independent variables (e.g., smoking status, gender, age) may be defining subgroups for which there are no outcomes. For example it may be that among nonsmoking women under the age of forty-five years no heart attacks have occurred. Because this group has no members, the computer cannot determine the parameters for the variables of smoking status, gender, and age.

> **TIP**
>
> If your model does not converge even after increasing the number of iterations, try decreasing the number of independent variables in your model.

What can you do if your model won't converge and your outcome variable is correctly coded? You should check to see if your independent variables define any subgroups with no outcomes. If this is not the case, you may be able to increase the number of attempts (iterations) the program makes to solve the equation. However, beware that if the equation is not solved with the default criteria of the number of iterations, there may be an inherent problem with your model. Try decreasing the number of independent variables in your model so that there are no subgroups with very few outcomes. Removing independent variables that have very skewed distributions, especially less than 5 percent of subjects in a particular category, usually helps the most.

Interpreting the results

8.1 What information will my multivariable analysis produce?

Multivariable techniques produce two major kinds of information: Information about how well the model (all the independent variables together) fit the data and information about the relationship of each of the independent variables to the outcome variable (with adjustment for all other independent variables in the analysis). In this chapter, we will review information that is routinely output from multivariable software programs. In the next chapter we will delve deeper into how well the assumptions of the models are fulfilled and how to improve the fit of the models by looking at supplementary techniques that you may request.

8.2 How do I assess how well my model fits the data?

Although there is some overlap, the methods for determining how well a model accounts for the outcome differ by type of multivariable analysis (Table 8.1). The methods for each model are discussed below.

8.2.A Multiple linear regression

We start the assessment of a multiple linear regression model by testing whether the independent variables predict the outcome better than assuming that everyone in the study had the mean value for the outcome.[1] If knowing the values of the independent variables improves the fit more than would be expected by chance, then the value of F will be large. A large F value for a given

---

[1] Within ANOVA, the F test has an analogous meaning. However, because multiple linear regression is performed more commonly than ANOVA in clinical research with interval variables, and because I want to keep the prose of this section simple, I will refer only to multiple linear regression. To see how to set up the same analysis using either ANOVA or multiple linear regression and how the F test is calculated for each see: Glantz, S. A. and Slinker, B. K. *Primer of Applied Regression & Analysis of Variance*. 2nd edn. New York, NY: McGraw-Hill, 2001, pp. 294–302.

Table 8.1 Methods for assessing how well a model accounts for the outcome.

	Multiple linear regression	Multiple (binary) logistic regression	Proportional odds regression	Multinomial logistic regression	Proportional hazards analysis	Poisson regression (negative binomial regression)
Independent variables are associated with outcome more than would be expected by chance	F test	Likelihood ratio test	Likelihood ratio test	Likelihood ratio test	Likelihood ratio test	Likelihood ratio test
Quantitative/ qualitative assessment of how well model accounts for outcome	R^{2*}	Pearson goodness-of-fit Deviance goodness-of-fit Comparison of estimated to observed value Hosmer–Lemeshow test* Sensitivity, specificity, accuracy (requires choosing a cut-off) c index*	c index Create separate binary models and use same statistics as with binary logistic regression.	Create separate binary models and use same statistics as with binary logistic regression.	Comparison of estimated to observed outcome.	Deviance goodness-of-fit test*

* Best tests/most commonly reported tests are shown with an asterisk.

sample size and a given number of variables in the model (which determines the degrees of freedom) will result in a small P value. This indicates that the null hypothesis of no association between the independent variables and the outcome can be rejected.

A major limitation of the F test is that it does not tell you which or how many variables in your model are significant. You can have a model with five variables in it, four of which are unassociated with the outcome, and still have a significant overall test. Methods for determining the statistical significance of the individual variables are dealt with in Section 8.3.

Another limitation is that knowing that the variables as a group are more closely associated with outcome than you would expect by chance does not tell

> A major limitation of the F test is that it does not tell you which or how many variables in your model are significant.

TIP

If individual variables are significantly related to outcome but your overall model is not statistically significant, delete those variables that are not associated with outcome.

you quantitatively how well your independent variables account for outcome. Given these limitations, what is this test useful for? If you get a global F test that is not significant, you should worry that your model is a poor representation of your data. If individual variables are significantly related to outcome, and the overall model is not statistically significant, it suggests that there are many variables included in the model that are unrelated to outcome. Consider deleting variables from your model that are not associated with outcome.

The R^2 is generally more useful than the F test because it provides a quantitative measure of how well the independent variables explain the outcome. The R^2, also called the coefficient of variation, indicates how much better you can account for the outcome by knowing the values of the independent variables than by assuming that everyone had the mean value on the outcome variable.

DEFINITION

R^2 is a quantitative measure of how well the independent variables account for the outcome.

TIP

When R^2 is multiplied by 100 it can be thought of as the percentage of the variance in the dependent variable explained by the independent variables.

The value of R^2 ranges from 0 (indicating that the independent variables do not explain the outcome any better than assuming everyone has the sample mean) to 1 (the independent variables completely account for the outcome). When R^2 is multiplied by 100 it can be thought of as the percentage of the variance in the dependent variable explained by the independent variables.

While R^2 is generally more informative than F, it has the limitation that its value will increase as you include additional independent variables, even if these variables add only a little bit of information. For example, a model with ten independent variables will have a higher R^2 than a model with five of these variables, even if the additional five variables add little to the model. To account for this, the statistic-adjusted R^2 charges you a price for each variable in your model. As you add variables, adjusted R^2 can increase (the gain in having the variable is greater than the charge), decrease (the charge is greater than the gain), or stay the same (the gain and the charge are equal).

Adjusted R^2 charges you a price for each variable in your model.

8.2.B   Multiple logistic regression

Use the likelihood ratio test to assess the fit of a logistic regression model.

With multiple (binary) logistic regression the likelihood ratio test (often referred to as model chi-squared) is used to test whether the independent variables are associated with outcome more than would be expected by chance. It is analogous to the F test but has a chi-squared distribution. If knowing the values of the independent variables predicts the outcome better than assuming the mean outcome for the subjects (in the case of a dichotomous outcome the mean is simply the proportion of persons who experience an outcome), and this improvement is more than you would expect by chance, then the value of the chi-squared associated with the likelihood ratio will be large.

When the chi-squared of the likelihood ratio test is large, the *P* value will be small and the null hypothesis can be rejected.

When the chi-squared of the likelihood ratio test is large, for a given number of parameters in the model (degrees of freedom), the *P* value will be small. As with a large F test value, you will reject the null hypothesis and conclude that the independent variables are related to the outcome. The *P* value associated with the chi-squared assumes a "large" sample size; sample sizes greater than 80–100 give a good approximation.[2]

In addition to the likelihood ratio test, software programs will routinely calculate two goodness-of-fit statistics: Pearson and deviance. The statistics compare observed and expected values from the model, with a high value indicating a lack of fit. The tests produce *P* values calculated from a chi-squared distribution, which is generally appropriate for these tests.[3]

TIP

A useful qualitative method for assessing a logistic regression model is to compare the estimated probability of outcome to the observed probability of outcome.

The Hosmer–Lemeshow test is a better test of goodness of fit. The statistic compares the estimated to observed likelihood of outcome for groups of subjects. To appreciate the basis of this test, recall that the estimated probability of outcome is based on the pattern of independent variables for each subject. If your model has three variables, gender (male/female), age (in terciles), and hypertension (yes/no), then the number of distinct patterns of these three variables is $2 \times 3 \times 2 = 12$. In other words, whether you have 15 subjects or 15 million there are only 12 distinct patterns. For each of these patterns, there is an observed rate of outcome (the proportion of persons who experienced the outcome based on the data) and an estimated rate of outcome (based on the model).

The Hosmer–Lemeshow test is based on dividing the sample into approximately ten groups based on the range of estimated probability of outcome (the first group contains the ten percent of subjects with the lowest estimated likelihood of outcome, the second group contains the ten percent of subjects with the next-lowest estimated likelihood of outcome, etc.). In a well-fitting model, the estimated likelihood will be close to the observed likelihood of outcome. This will result in a small chi-squared and a non-significant *P* value.

DEFINITION

The *Hosmer–Lemeshow goodness-of-fit test* compares the estimated to observed likelihood of outcome for groups of subjects.

From this explanation, you can appreciate that the Hosmer–Lemeshow test is essentially a summary of how well the estimated values of a logistic model fit the observed values. Rather than obtain a summary, it is often useful to directly compare the estimated probability of outcome (according to

---

[2] For a more detailed explanation of the likelihood ratio test, see: Hosmer, D. W. and Lemeshow, S. *Applied Logistic Regression.* New York, NY: Wiley, 1989, pp. 8–18; Menard, S. *Applied Logistic Regression Analysis.* Thousand Oaks, CA: Sage Publications, 1995, pp. 19–21.

[3] Harrell, F. E. *Regression Modeling Strategies: With applications to linear models, logistic regression, and survival analysis.* New York: Springer, 2001, p.231; Kluss, O. "Global goodness-of-fit tests in logistic regression with sparse data." At http://oliverkuss.de/science/publications/Kuss_Poster_Global_Goodness-of-fit_Tests_in_Logistic_Regression_with_Sparse_Data.pdf.

the model) to the observed probability of outcome (the original data) using a tabular or graphic form.

If you have a large number of distinct covariate patterns, you may need to group subjects with similar estimated likelihood of outcomes together. Thus, for example, you may divide your sample into ten groups of estimated likelihood of outcome: 0–0.10, 0.11–0.20, etc. If you have a few persons who have very high or very low estimated probabilities of outcome and you group subjects into equal divisions of likelihood of outcome, you may still have very small groups. An alternative is to divide the probabilities such that there are approximately equal numbers of outcomes in each group.

For example, Gordon and colleagues evaluated racial variation in predicted and observed in-hospital death rates.[4] The investigators used logistic regression to develop an estimated probability of in-hospital death. They included in their model age, sex, race, type of health insurance, emergency department admission, and a mortality measure based on data from the first 48 hours of hospitalization. They divided the estimated risk of death into ten strata so that there would be equal numbers of outcomes in each group (653–654 deaths). Note that since the strata are based on the number of outcomes rather than the estimated risk of death, the different strata have varying widths of estimated risks of death (stratum 1 ranges from only 0.00 to 0.03, whereas stratum 10 ranges from 0.81 to 1.00). You can see that the estimated risk of death was similar to the observed probability of death in the ten strata (Table 8.2).

Although the authors published their data in tabular form, qualitative assessments of the fit of a logistic model can sometimes be better appreciated in graphic form. For example, I have created Figure 8.1 by plotting the midpoint of the estimated probability of death on the x-axis against the observed probability of death along the y-axis for a study of racial variation in hospital death. You can see that the points (connected by a solid line) are all close to the dotted diagonal line, which represents perfect calibration.

If the points fall close to the diagonal, as in Figure 8.1, your model is an excellent estimate of outcome. If the points are scattered far from the line, it indicates that the model is not very accurate at estimating observed outcomes. An advantage of this approach is that it also allows you to see if your model performs better at certain probabilities of disease.

Another way to assess the fit of a model is to quantify how well it predicts the outcome of study subjects. To do this you must dichotomize the estimated

[4] Gordon, H.S., Harper, D.L., and Rosenthal, G.E. "Racial variation in predicted and observed in-hospital death." *JAMA* **276** (1996): 1639–44.

Table 8.2 Comparison of estimated to observed risk of death among hospitalized patients.

Stratum	Estimated risk of death	Observed risk of death
1	0.00–0.03	0.01
2	0.03–0.06	0.05
3	0.06–0.10	0.09
4	0.10–0.17	0.14
5	0.17–0.24	0.24
6	0.24–0.34	0.32
7	0.34–0.47	0.38
8	0.47–0.63	0.52
9	0.63–0.81	0.66
10	0.81–1.00	0.87

Adapted with permission from Gordon, H. S., *et al.* "Racial variation in predicted and observed in-hospital death." *JAMA* **276** (1996): 1639–44. Copyright 1996, American Medical Association.

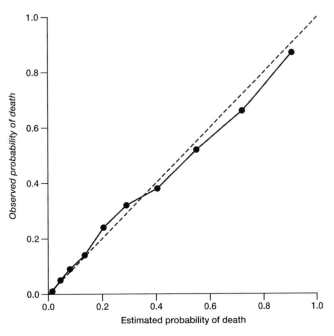

Figure 8.1   Estimated (*x*-axis) versus observed values (*y*-axis) for risk of death among hospitalized patients. The dotted diagonal line represents perfect calibration. Data from Gordon, H. S., *et al.* "Racial variation in predicted and observed in-hospital death." *JAMA* **276** (1996): 1639–44.

outcome. In other words, you must choose a cut-off of what estimated probability of outcome you will consider to be a prediction of outcome. Once you do this, you can compute the sensitivity (proportion of persons who are predicted to have the outcome who really have it), specificity (proportion of persons who do not have the outcome who are predicted not to have it), and the proportion of correctly identified persons.

Choosing the cut-off for probability of outcome is not always easy. Each cut-off has a different sensitivity, specificity, and proportion of correctly identified persons. One simple cut-off is to assume that anyone with probability of outcome greater than 50 percent is predicted to have the outcome. However, the choice of 0.5 as the cut-off for measuring the predictive ability of your model may not be best. This is especially true for clinical diseases (e.g., ischemic heart disease) where even relatively low probabilities of disease are worrisome because of the seriousness of the disease. For example it would not be appropriate to send a patient with chest pain home who had a 49 percent probability of having acute ischemia. For this reason, models predicting acute ischemia choose a much lower cut-off, such as seven percent for computing sensitivity and specificity.[5]

> **DEFINITION**
>
> The *c index* is a measure of the concordance between predicted and observed outcomes. The higher the value the greater the ability of your model to predict outcome.

Another useful measure of how well your logistic regression model predicts outcome is the c index.[6] It is a measure of the concordance between predicted and observed outcomes. Here's how it works: In any data set there will be pairs of subjects who have the same observed outcome (e.g., both have had heart attacks, neither have had heart attacks) and some who have different outcomes (e.g., one had a heart attack, one did not). For each pair of subjects with different outcomes, one can ask whether the model predicts a higher likelihood of outcome for the subject in the pair who experiences the outcome or for the subject who does not experience the outcome. If the subject with the higher predicted likelihood of outcome actually experiences the outcome the pair is concordant (with outcome). If the case with the higher predicted likelihood of outcome does not have the outcome, the pair is discordant. If the model predicts the same probability of outcome for both cases, the pair is tied. The c index equals the proportion of concordant cases plus half of the ties. A value of 0.5 would indicate that the model does not discriminate any better than chance. The higher the c value is (maximum 1) the greater the ability of your model to predict outcome.

[5] Goldman, L., Cook, E. F., Brand, D. A., *et al.* "A computer protocol to predict myocardial infarction in emergency department patients with chest pain." *N. Engl. J. Med.* **318** (1988): 797–803.

[6] Harrell, F. E., Lee, K. L., Matchar, D. B., *et al.* "Regression models for prognostic prediction: Advantages, problems, and suggested solutions." *Cancer Treat. Rep.* **69** (1985): 1071–7.

Although there is an R^2 measure for logistic regression, it does not perform as well for this type of analysis as it does for multiple linear regression and is rarely reported in the literature.

8.2.C Proportional odds regression model

Proportional odds regression, as with (binary) multiple logistic regression, generates a likelihood ratio test. A significant P value indicates that you can reject the null hypothesis that the independent variables are unassociated with outcome. However, the test has the same limitations as with binary multiple logistic regression: it does not tell you which variables are associated with outcome nor how strongly the variables are associated with outcome, just that the association is more than you would expect by chance.

As with (binary) multiple logistic regression it is possible to calculate a c statistic. The higher the c value the greater the ability of your model to predict outcome.

To get a better sense of the fit of a proportional odds logistic regression model, you can create separate binary logistic models (the number of models would be one less than the number of levels of the outcome variable). For each model the program will calculate the same statistics that you would have with a binary logistic model (e.g., Hosmer–Lemeshow test, c test). If each of the individual models fit well, it is likely that the overall proportional odds model also fits well.[7]

> **TIP**
>
> Use the score test to assess the proportional odds assumption.

8.2.D Multinomial logistic regression

Multinomial logistic regression also generates a likelihood ratio test that when significant tells you that you can reject the null hypothesis that the independent variables are unassociated with outcome.

To get a better sense of the fit of a multinomial logistic regression model, you can create separate binary logistic models (the number of models would be one less than the number of groups of the outcome variable).[8] Each binary logistic model compares the reference group chosen for the multinomial logistic regression model to one of the other groups. For each model the program will calculate the same statistics that would be generated with a binary logistic model (e.g., Hosmer–Lemeshow test, c test). If each of the individual models

[7] For more on this strategy see: Hosmer, D. W. and Lemeshow, S. *Applied Logistic Regression*. 2nd edn. New York: John Wiley, pp. 305–8

[8] For more on this strategy see: Hosmer, D. W. and Lemeshow, S. *Applied Logistic Regression*. 2nd edn. New York: John Wiley, pp. 280–7.

fit well, it is likely that the overall multinomial logistic regression model also fits well.

8.2.E Proportional hazards analysis

As with logistic regression analysis, the likelihood ratio test is used to assess whether the independent variables are associated with the outcome. If the time to outcome of subjects with certain values on their independent variables are different from the baseline rate (more than you would expect by chance) then the chi-squared associated with the likelihood ratio test will be statistically significant.

It is also possible to compare estimated and observed time to outcome. This can be done using Kaplan–Meier survival curves for each important subgroup of patients defined by your model. For example, Colford and colleagues found in their proportional hazards analysis that two variables, CD4 count and hematocrit (both split at the median), had the strongest association with survival among HIV-infected patients with cryptosporidiosis.[9] To assess how well their model estimated survival, they stratified their patients into four groups based on CD4 count and hematocrit. As shown in Table 8.3, they found that the estimated and observed median survival times were similar.

Because the underlying survival function is not automatically estimated in proportional hazards analysis, you need to use adjunct estimators to calculate estimated median survival. Also, this procedure will not work if there are few subjects who experienced the outcome. (To calculate an estimated median survival, half of the sample for each covariate pattern must experience the outcome.)

8.2.F Poisson regression and negative binomial regression

> If the Poisson distribution fits the data, the deviance divided by the degrees of freedom should have a value of about 1.

To assess the fit of a Poisson or negative binomial regression model, report the likelihood ratio test.[10] If the test is significant then the independent variables are associated with outcome more than would be expected by chance.

To determine whether the Poisson distribution fits the data, look at the deviance goodness-of-fit test. The value of the deviance divided by the degrees

[9] Colford, J. M., Tager, I. B., Hirozawa, A. M., *et al.* "Cryptosporidiosis among patients infected with human immunodeficiency virus: Factors related to symptomatic infection and survival." *Am. J. Epidemiol.* **144** (1996): 807–16.

[10] This test is also referred to as the deviance test statistic. I prefer likelihood ratio to distinguish it from the deviance goodness-of-fit test. See: "Poisson Regression" at: www.statsdirect.com/help/regression_and_correlation?poisson_regression.htm.

Table 8.3 Survival among subgroups of HIV-infected patients with *Cryptosporidium*.

Subgroup	Relative hazard	95% confidence interval	Median survival (days)	
			Estimated	Observed
CD4 count ≤53 cells/ml and hematocrit ≤37%	15.9	6.0–42.2	213	204
CD4 count ≤53 cells/ml and hematocrit > 37%	8.1	2.8–23.6	465	341
CD4 count >53 cells/ml and hematocrit ≤37%	3.1	1.1–8.8	688	878
CD4 count >53 cells/ml and hematocrit > 37%	1.0 (ref.)		1,119	1,119

Adapted with permission from Colford, J. M., *et al.* "Cryptosporidiosis among patients infected with human immunodeficiency virus." *Am. J. Epidemiol.* **144** (1996): 807–16.

of freedom (this may be output as Deviance Value/df) should have a value of about 1 if the data fit a Poisson distribution. In this case, the *P* value will be non-significant. On the other hand, if the value of the deviance divided by the degrees of freedom is much larger than one and the *P* value is statistically significant, the data may be overdispersed, in which case you should retry the model using a negative binomial distribution.

8.3 What do the coefficients tell me about the relationship between each variable and the outcome?

DEFINITION

A variable's *coefficient* tells you how the modeled outcome changes with a one-unit change in the independent variable.

With multivariable analysis a variable's coefficient (also called beta) tells you how the outcome changes with changes in the independent variable, while adjusting for the other independent variables in the model. Coefficients can be positive or negative. Because the different multivariable techniques are modeling different outcomes, there are differences in how these coefficients are interpreted (Table 8.4).

8.3.A Coefficients in multiple linear regression[11]

In multiple linear regression, the mean value of the outcome is modeled (Table 8.4). For each increase (decrease) in the independent variable, the mean

[11] Strictly speaking, ANOVA does not produce regression coefficients and therefore I have not listed it in the title of the subsection. However, when you perform an ANOVA analysis your printout may well show you regression coefficients. These coefficients are based on a linear regression approach to the problem. As explained in Section 3.2.D, ANOVA and linear regression produce the same results if set up in the same way.

Table 8.4 Meaning of individual variable coefficients from multivariable models.

Multivariable technique	What is being modeled?	What does coefficient mean?	Special meaning of coefficient
Multiple linear regression	Mean value of the outcome	For each increase (decrease) in the independent variable, the mean value of the outcome increases (decreases) by the amount of the coefficient	Coefficient = slope of line describing the relationship of the independent variable to the outcome
Multiple (binary) logistic regression	The logarithm of the odds (the logit) of the outcome	For each increase (decrease) in the independent variable, the logit of the outcome increases (decreases) by the amount of the coefficient	Exponentiated coefficient = odds ratio ($e^{coefficient}$ = odds ratio); odds ratio is the likelihood of having the outcome compared to not having the outcome
Proportional odds regression	Cumulative logit of the outcome	For each increase (decrease) in the independent variable, the logit for going from one level to the next level of the outcome increases (decreases) by the amount of the coefficient.	Exponentiated coefficient = odds ratio ($e^{coefficient}$ = odds ratio); odds ratio is the likelihood of being in one level of the outcome compared to being in the next level of the outcome
Multinomial logistic regression	Logit of being in one category of the outcome versus the reference category of the outcome	For each increase (decrease) in the independent variable, the logit of being in a particular category compared to the reference group increases (decreases) by the amount of the coefficient	Exponentiated coefficient = odds ratio ($e^{coefficient}$ = odds ratio); odds ratio is the likelihood of being in one category compared to the reference category
Proportional hazards analysis	The logarithm of the relative hazard	For each increase (decrease) in the independent variable, the logarithm of the relative hazard increases (decreases) the amount of the coefficient	Exponentiated coefficient = relative hazard ($e^{coefficient}$ = relative hazard); relative hazard is the likelihood of having the outcome versus not having the outcome
Poisson regression and negative binomial regression	The logarithm of the outcome	For each increase (decrease) in the independent variable, the logarithm of the outcome increases (decreases) by the amount of the coefficient	Exponentiated coefficient = relative risk (or relative incidence) ($e^{coefficient}$ = relative risk); relative risk is how much higher the count or rate is with a one-unit change in the independent variable

value of the outcome increases (decreases) by the amount of the coefficient. A positive coefficient indicates that the independent variable and the outcome variable are moving (up or down) together. A negative coefficient indicates that the independent variable and the dependent variable are moving in opposite directions.

For example, let's say that you are assessing the association between the age (measured in years) and the outcome variable, cholesterol level (measured in mg/dl), with statistical adjustment for dietary intake of cholesterol. In your multiple linear regression model, the adjusted coefficient for age is 0.2. The units for the coefficient would be mg/(dl year). This means that for each year the mean cholesterol value increases by 0.2 mg/dl. If the coefficient were –0.2, it would mean that for each year the mean cholesterol value decreases by 0.2 mg/dl.

> With linear regression, the coefficient equals the slope of the line.

With linear regression, the coefficient has a special property: it is the slope of the line describing the relationship of the independent variable to the outcome. With the slope and one point you can draw a line showing the best estimated value for all possible values of your dependent variable. One point which the software program will automatically output is the intercept (the point on the y-axis where x is zero).

For each coefficient of your multiple linear regression model your software program will calculate a P value. The P value is based on a t test, where t is

$$t = \frac{\text{coefficient}}{\text{standard error}}$$

> If the coefficient is much bigger than the error associated with estimating the coefficient, the t value will be large and the P value will be small and statistically significant.

The t value has an intuitive meaning. If the coefficient is much bigger than the error associated with estimating the coefficient, the t value will be large and the P value will be small and statistically significant. Indeed, t values greater than 2.0 (coefficient is two times the standard error) are statistically significant at the traditional $P < 0.05$ value (as long as the degrees of freedom are at least 60). When the P value is statistically significant, we reject the hypothesis that the coefficient is zero (which is equivalent to saying the slope of the line is zero, or that the line is horizontal).

8.3.B Coefficient in multiple (binary) logistic regression

The meaning of the coefficient in logistic regression is different from its meaning in linear regression because logistic regression is modeling the logarithm of the odds of the outcome; this is known as the logit (Table 8.4). With logistic regression the coefficient tells you how a one-unit change in the independent variable changes the logit. A positive coefficient means that as the variable increases, the logit increases. A negative coefficient means that as the variable increases, the logit decreases.

To interpret the meaning of the coefficients in logistic regression, you must know which value of the outcome the logit is estimating. The default on most software programs is to determine the logit for the lower numerical value (determined by how you have coded your variables). But you could ask the computer to determine the logit of the higher numerical value. Either way, the results would be the same but the signs of the coefficients would be different. Make sure you know for which value of your outcome variable the computer is estimating the logit.

TIP

Make sure you know for which value of your outcome variable the computer is estimating the logit.

The coefficients in logistic regression have a special meaning. If you exponentiate (take the antilogarithm of) the coefficient, you will obtain the odds ratio. This is simply the mathematical constant e raised to the power of the coefficient's value:

$$\text{odds ratio} = e^{\text{coefficient}}$$

Although your statistical program will output the odds ratio automatically, if you needed to calculate it yourself from the coefficient simply enter the coefficient in your calculator, add a negative sign if the coefficient is negative and press the button with the little *e* on it. If your calculator has no *e* button, buy a new calculator or use Excel (the 'exp' function).

DEFINITION

The *odds ratio* is equal to the antilogarithm of the coefficient from logistic regression.

The odds ratio tells you how much the likelihood of the outcome changes with a one-unit change in the independent variable. When the odds ratio is greater than 1 then the risk of the outcome increases as an independent variable increases or when a dichotomous independent variable is yes/present (assuming it is coded 1 = yes/present and 0 = no/absent). When the odds ratio is less than 1 then the risk of the outcome decreases as an interval-independent variable increases or when a dichotomous independent variable is yes/present (assuming it is coded 1 = yes/present and 0 = no/absent). An odds ratio of 1 indicates that there is no change in the likelihood of outcome with changes in the independent variable.

In published work, you will see many other terms used for the odds ratio including relative risk, risk, and risk ratio. The odds ratio is the preferred term because it will alert your reader that you have used logistic regression. Odds ratios approximate the relative risk, but only when the outcome is uncommon (<15 percent). However, even when the outcome is common, it is okay to report the odds ratio as long as you are clear that it does not equal the relative risk.

To assess the precision of the odds ratios you will want to calculate the 95% confidence intervals. They are easily obtained by the extension of the formula for computing the odds ratio. Your statistical packages will auto-matically compute the confidence intervals, but it is handy to know how to calculate it, in case you ever need to. To obtain the upper confidence interval use the addition sign; to obtain the lower confidence interval use the subtrac-tion sign. The standard error is usually next to the coefficient on the computer printout.

$$95\% \text{ confidence interval for odds ratio} = e^{\text{coefficient} \pm 1.96 \text{ (standard error)}}$$

Looking at the formula you can also see how the precision of the estimate (measured by the standard error) is reflected in the confidence intervals. If the standard error is large you will be adding (or subtracting) a large number from the coefficient. This will result in the upper limit being much bigger than the odds ratio/relative hazard and the lower limit being much smaller than the odds ratio/relative hazard.

Of course, you don't have to use 95 percent confidence intervals. For some exploratory studies you may wish to report 90 percent confidence intervals. For other studies, where precision is very important, you may wish to report 99 percent confidence intervals. The formula is the same as the one shown above except that instead of 1.96, which is the standard normal deviate for 95 percent confidence intervals, you substitute the standard normal deviate for the confidence intervals you want (1.66 for 90 percent confidence intervals; 2.576 for 99 percent confidence intervals).

You will also want to know whether the coefficients (and by extensions the odds ratios) are statistically significant. To do this use the Wald test. It is based on either the chi-squared or the z distribution:

$$\frac{\text{chi-squared}}{\text{distribution}} = \left\{ \frac{\text{coefficient}}{\text{standard error}} \right\}^2 \text{ or } \frac{z}{\text{distribution}} = \frac{\text{coefficient}}{\text{standard error}}$$

TIP

Use the Wald chi-squared for testing the significance of individual coefficients from logistic regression.

With either formula, coefficients that are twice their standard error will be significant at $P < 0.05$. The Wald test assumes a large sample size (i.e., 80–100 or more subjects).

There are two other tests that you can use to determine the statistical signifi-cance of a particular coefficient: the likelihood ratio test and the score test.[12]

---

[12] You met the likelihood ratio test in Section 8.2.B on evaluating whether your model accounts for outcome better than chance. The difference is that here you are comparing models with a particu-lar variable present to models where that variable is absent (but the other independent variables are present). In Section 8.2.B this test compared models that contained all of the independent variables to models that contained none of the independent variables.

Table 8.5 Output from a multiple logistic regression model of the relationship between individual variables and favorable neurologic outcome.

	Coefficient	Standard error	Wald chi-squared	P value	Odds ratio	95% confidence interval
Age (per year)	−0.020	0.005	16.32	0.0001	0.98	0.96–0.99
Cardiac cause vs. no cardiac cause	0.802	0.581	1.90	0.16	2.23	0.72 – 6.96
Time from collapse to first bystander resuscitation attempt (min)	−0.051	0.051	1.01	0.31	0.95	0.86–1.05
Cardiac-only resuscitation vs. conventional CPR	0.798	0.327	5.94	0.01	2.22	1.17– 4.21
Time from first bystander resuscitation attempt to first AED analysis (min)	−0.287	0.076	14.43	0.0001	0.75	0.65– 0.87
Ventricular fibrillation or pulseless ventricular tachycardia vs. other rhythm	2.079	0.425	23.9	0.0001	8.00	3.48–18.41

The likelihood ratio test is based on comparing the likelihood when the variable is not in the model to the likelihood when the variable is in the model. To compute the test statistic for models where you have multiple independent variables, each variable is singly dropped while retaining the other variables in the model. The statistic follows a chi-squared distribution. Computation of the score test is based on derivatives of the likelihood ratio. It also follows a chi-squared distribution.

Although there are situations when the likelihood ratio test may perform better,[13] most researchers use the Wald chi-squared. If your results are robust you should get similar results with all three tests.

To better understand the meaning of coefficients in logistic regression (and because it will also help in understanding the coefficients from proportional odds regression, multinomial regression, proportional hazards analysis, Poisson and negative binomial regression), look at Table 8.5. The data are from the observational study of chest compression only CPR discussed in Section 3.3.[14]

Column 1 shows the regression coefficient; column 2 shows the standard error of the regression coefficient, column 3 shows the Wald chi-squared,

TIP

If you code your outcome in the opposite direction, the coefficients will stay the same but the sign will change. If you don't keep track of how your variables are coded you will not correctly interpret your analysis.

[13] Hauck, W. W. and Donner, A. "Wald's test as applied to hypotheses in logit analysis." *J. Am. Stat. Assoc.* **72** (1977): 851–3.
[14] SOS-Kanto Study Group. "Cardiopulmonary resuscitation by bystanders with chest compression only (SOS-Kanto): An observational study." *Lancet* **369** (2007): 920–6.

column 4 shows the *P* value of the Wald chi-squared, column 5 shows the odds ratio, and column 6 shows the 95% confidence interval for the odds ratio.

Looking first at the coefficients in column 1, we see that certain coefficients are positive and certain coefficients are negative. When the coefficient is positive the logit of the outcome (in this case a favorable neurologic outcome) increases as the independent variable increases or when a dichotomous independent variable is yes/present (assuming variable is coded as 1 = yes/present and 0 = no/absent). Therefore having a cardiac cause of the arrest (row 2), would make a favorable neurologic outcome more likely (assuming that the variable is coded cardiac cause yes = 1 and no = 0). When the coefficient is negative, the logit of the outcome decreases as the independent variable increases or when a dichotomous independent variable is yes/present (assuming variable is coded as 1 = yes/present and 0 = no/absent). Therefore as age increases (row 1) a favorable neurologic outcome is less likely.

If the outcome were coded such that we were predicting an unfavorable neurologic outcome, the coefficients would be the same but the signs would be in the opposite direction. Similarly, if the variable in row 2 were coded as no cardiac cause = 1 vs. cardiac cause = 0, the coefficient would be the same, but the sign would be in the opposite direction. I hope you can appreciate why I took you so laboriously through the issue of coding of variables in Section 7.1. If you don't keep track of how your variables are coded you will not correctly interpret your analysis.

A second critical lesson from Table 8.5 is that the size of the coefficient does not allow you to compare the variables and determine which one is most strongly associated with the outcome unless all the variables are in the same units and have the same level of precision. Said in the opposite way: the size of the coefficient hinges on the units it is measured in and its precision reflects the size of the standard error. To illustrate, if you look at column 1, you see that the coefficient for age (–0.020) is the smallest of all the coefficients. But this is not because age has the weakest association with neurologic outcome; it is because age is measured in single years. If age were measured in 10 years, the coefficient would be –0.20 or 10 times bigger. That's because if the coefficient associated with 1 year were –0.02 then the coefficient associated with 10 years would be –0.02 + –0.02 +–0.02 +–0.02 +–0.02 –0.02 + –0.02 +–0.02 +–0.02 +–0.02 or –0.20. Looking back at Table 8.5 you can appreciate that for a 10-year period, age would no longer be the smallest coefficient; however, grouping the units in 10-year bands in no way changes the importance of a variable.

Another interesting aspect of the variable age is how small the standard error is relative to the coefficient. That's probably because age – compared to many

> **TIP**
>
> The importance of a coefficient depends not on its size but on the units it is measured in and the size of its standard error.

other variables – can be measured with more precision and is more likely to be accurate in observational medical records. Because the standard error is very small, the Wald test for the variable age is one of the largest even though the coefficient for age is one of the smallest. A large value of the Wald test, yields a small P value. Compare the variable age to the variable time from collapse to first bystander resuscitation attempt in minutes. Although the coefficient for the latter variable is larger than for age, the standard error is as big as the coefficient. Given that, it is no surprise that the coefficient is not statistically significant.

Those coefficients with a positive sign yield odds ratios that are greater than one, while those with a negative sign yield odds ratios less than one. In studies such as this, where the outcome is uncommon (only 5% of subjects with any type of bystander resuscitation had a favorable neurologic outcome) the odds ratios tell you how the likelihood of the outcome changes with a one-unit change of the independent variable. So a 1-year increase in age (odds ratio = 0.98) is associated with a 2% decrease in the likelihood of favorable neurologic outcome. Conversely receiving cardiac-only resuscitation (odds ratio = 2.2) more than doubles (multiplies by 2.2) the chance of a favorable neurologic outcome.

To determine the impact of a multiple unit change, you would take the odds ratio to the power of the number of units of change. For example, a 10-year increase in age would be associated with an odds ratio equal to $(0.98)^{12}$ or 0.82. (You may be surprised that to determine the coefficient for a multiple unit change you add the coefficients for a single unit change, and that to determine the odds ratio for a multiple unit changes you multiply odds ratio. To prove to yourself that this is correct, exponentiate the coefficient for a 10-unit change of age [−0.20] and you will get an odds ratio of 0.82.)

Looking back at the formula for calculating the 95% confidence intervals for the odds ratios, you will appreciate that if the standard error is large compared to the coefficient, then the confidence intervals will be wide; this is the case for the variable of arrest owing to a cardiac cause. Wide confidence intervals may signify error in measurement, insufficient sample size, or skewed distribution of the independent variable.

8.3.C Coefficients in proportional odds regression

Since proportional odds regression is an extension of logistic regression, there are many similarities in the meaning of the coefficients. For example, the

> The odds ratio of proportional odds regression tells you how the likelihood of going from one level of the outcome variable to the next level of the outcome variable changes with a change in the independent variable.

exponentiated coefficient is also equal to the odds ratio, and the 95% confidence intervals and the *P* values are calculated in the same way. The major difference is that with binary logistic regression the logit of the outcome is being modeled while with proportional odds regression it is the **cumulative** logit of the outcome that is being modeled (Table 8.4). Therefore, the odds ratio of proportional odds regression tells you how the likelihood of going from one level of the outcome variable to the next level of the outcome variable changes with a change in the independent variable.

When the odds ratio is greater than 1 then the likelihood of the outcome going from one level to the next level increases as the independent variable increases or when a dichotomous independent variable is yes/present (assuming it is coded 1 = yes/present and 0 = no/absent). When the odds ratio is less then one then the likelihood of the outcome going from one level to the next level decreases as an interval-independent variable increases or when a dichotomous independent variable is yes/present (assuming it is coded 1 = yes/present and 0 = no/absent). As with binary logistic regression, the odds ratio only approximates the relative risk when the outcome is uncommon.

8.3.D Coefficients in multinomial logistic regression

With multinomial logistic regression the exponentiated coefficient is equal to the odds ratio and the 95% confidence intervals and the *P* values are calculated just as they are with binary logistic or proportional odds regression. However, multinomial logistic regression is modeling the logit of being in one category of the outcome compared to being in the reference category (Table 8.4). Therefore, the odds ratio of multinomial regression tells you how the likelihood of being in one category versus being in the reference group changes with a change in the independent variable.

When the odds ratio is greater than 1 then the likelihood of being in one category versus being in the reference group increases as an interval-independent variable increases or when a dichotomous independent variable is yes/present (assuming it is coded 1 = yes/present and 0 = no/absent). When the odds ratio is less than one then the likelihood of being in one category versus being in the reference group decreases when an interval-independent variable increases or when a dichotomous independent variable is yes/present (assuming it is coded 1 = yes/present and 0 = no/absent). As with binary logistic regression and proportional odds regression, the odds ratio only approximates the relative risk when the outcome is uncommon.

8.3.E Coefficients in proportional hazards analysis

Proportional hazards analysis models the logarithm of the relative hazard. The coefficient tells you how much a one-unit change in the independent variable changes the logarithm of the relative hazard.

The meaning of the signs of the coefficients in proportional hazards analysis is similar to that in logistic regression. A positive coefficient indicates that as the independent variable increases, the logarithm of the relative hazard increases. A negative coefficient indicates that as the independent variable increases, the logarithm of the relative hazard decreases.

If you take the antilogarithm of the exponentiated coefficient of a proportional hazards analysis, you will obtain the relative hazard. The relative hazard is the ratio of time to outcome given a particular set of risk factors to time to outcome without these factors.

> **DEFINITION**
>
> The *relative hazard* is equal to the exponentiated coefficient from proportional hazards analysis.

Authors may refer to the relative hazard as a relative risk, risk ratio, rate ratio, and hazard ratio. However, relative hazard is the preferred term because it alerts your reader that you have performed proportional hazards analysis. The 95% confidence intervals and the *P* values for the relative hazard are calculated in the same way as with logistic regression.

When the relative hazard is greater than 1 then the risk of the outcome increases as an independent variable increases or when a dichotomous independent variable is yes/present (assuming it is coded 1 = yes/present and 0 = no/absent). When the relative hazard is less than 1 then the risk of the outcome decreases as an interval-independent variable increases or when a dichotomous independent variable is yes/present (assuming it is coded 1 = yes/present and 0 = no/absent).

8.3.F Coefficients in Poisson regression and negative binomial regression

Poisson regression and negative binomial regression model the logarithm of the outcome (Table 8.4). The coefficients tell you how much a one-unit change in the independent variable changes the logarithm of the outcome. The meaning of the signs of the coefficients is similar to that of the other types of multivariable analysis discussed in this chapter. A positive coefficient indicates that as the independent variable increases, the logarithm of the outcome increases. A negative coefficient indicates that as the independent variable increases, the logarithm of the outcome decreases.

With Poisson regression and negative binomial regression the exponentiated coefficient equals the relative risk (or relative incidence when comparing rates of developing a disease or condition). When the relative risk is greater than one then the risk of the outcome or rate of outcome increases as an independent variable increases or when a dichotomous independent variable is yes/present (assuming it is coded 1 = yes/present and 0 = no/absent). When the relative risk is less than 1 then the risk of the outcome decreases as an interval-independent variable increases or when a dichotomous independent variable is yes/present (assuming it is coded 1 = yes/present and 0 = no/absent).

As you would for an odds ratio or relative hazard, you will want to report the 95% confidence interval for the relative risk or relative incidence as well as the *P* value.

8.4 How do I interpret the results of interaction terms?

Having reviewed the meaning of coefficients, let's return to the question of how to interpret product terms used to represent interaction effects (Section 7.3). If the impact of the two variables together is substantially greater than the additive effect of the two variables, the coefficient will be positive and the associated *P* value will be statistically significant. If the impact of the two variables together is substantially less than the additive effect of the two variables, the coefficient will be negative and the associated *P* value will be statistically significant. If the impact of the two variables together is equal to the additive effect of the two variables, the coefficient will be close to zero and the associated *P* value will not be statistically significant.

8.5 Do I have to adjust my multivariable regression coefficients for multiple comparisons?

To answer this complicated question it is best to consider first the simpler case of bivariate analyses. Let's say, for example, that you are assessing the association of age (40–59 years, 60–79 years, 80–99 years) on cholesterol levels using analysis of variance. In addition to being interested in the comparison of the three groups, you are also interested in a pair-wise comparison of the youngest group to the oldest group. Intuitively, it makes sense that if you compare three groups, one group will be highest and one group will be lowest. Therefore, if you compare the highest and the lowest group, you are running a risk that you are capitalizing on chance. One way to deal with this issue is not to consider pair-wise comparisons unless the overall F (for the comparison of the three groups) is significant. In addition, you should set a more stringent cut-off for pair-wise comparisons before rejecting the null hypothesis. This is usually done using the Bonferroni correction. It "charges" you for the number of pair-wise comparisons by requiring a lower *P* value before concluding that a comparison is statistically significant. To calculate the correction, simply divide the usual *P* value (e.g., 0.05) by the number of pair-wise comparisons you are performing. If you are performing three pair-wise comparisons, you would reject the null hypothesis only if $P \leq 0.016$ ($0.05/3 = 0.016$).

When you perform multiple bivariate comparisons (for example, comparing two groups on 20 different variables), some statisticians also recommend adjusting for multiple comparisons. The theory is that, by chance, at least one of your 20 comparisons will be statistically significant at the $P < 0.05$ level (that's because $1/20 = 0.05$). However, instead, what most investigators do is perform a multivariable analysis. With multivariable analysis, you need not worry about multiple comparisons when performing tests of the significance of the overall model (F or likelihood ratio test). The reason is that you are performing only a single test to assess whether the independent variables (as a group) are associated with the outcome.

But when you turn to the question of whether the individual independent variables from your multivariable model are statistically associated with your outcome, you are essentially making multiple comparisons. As with bivariate comparisons, some statisticians advocate adjusting your *P* value for the number of independent variables in your model. If you have ten variables, you would require that the *P* value be < 0.005 ($0.05/10$) before concluding that the association between the independent variable and the outcome is significant.

However, there are major disadvantages to adjusting for multiple comparisons. They have been well articulated by the epidemiologist Kenneth Rothman.[15] He points out that the basis of adjustment for multiple comparisons is the assumption that chance is the most common explanation for an association between two things. But this assumption is flawed because the universe is governed by natural (physical) laws. Most associations in the universe have a true (rather than chance) connection. (Note that a true connection does not mean a causal connection.)

In addition, an individual comparison cannot "know" how many other comparisons you have made. Therefore an individual association cannot be more or less likely to be caused by chance based on how many other associations you have assessed. Rothman illustrates the absurdity of strict adherence to the principle of adjusting for multiple comparisons by asking: If you favor adjusting for multiple comparisons, should you adjust for the number of comparisons you assessed in a single paper, or the number of comparisons

---

[15] Rothman, K.J. "No adjustments are needed for multiple comparisons." *Epidemiology* **1** (1990): 43–6.

assessed in a series of papers analyzing the same data set, or the number of comparisons performed during your career?

Personally, I am swayed by Rothman's arguments and do not adjust for multiple comparisons with multivariable models. Nonetheless, if you are not going to adjust for multiple comparisons, there are measures that you should take to minimize potential problems. Tell your reader how many variables (comparisons) were tested in your analysis. Do not report only the independent variables that were significantly associated with outcome. Nonsignificant results, while much less sexy, are every bit as informative. Do not be a slave to the cut-off of $P < 0.05$, in either direction. Don't assume something is insignificant just because its P value is 0.06 or that something is significant just because its P value is 0.04. Use confidence intervals, whenever possible, instead of P values (although, as discussed above, confidence intervals are also subject to the potential multiple comparison problem, since they are based on the 95 percent probability that 95 percent of repeated samples of the population would produce 95 percent confidence intervals that would contain the true value). Most importantly, evaluate your findings in the light of previous work and biological plausibility. If you anticipate that a reviewer will not be convinced by the above, cite Rothman's article. It sometimes helps.[16]

[16] For more on the debate about multiple comparisons, see: Savitz, D. A. and Olshan, A. F. "Multiple comparisons and related issues in the interpretation of epidemiologic data." *Am. J. Epidemiol.* **142** (1995): 904–8; Thompson, J. "Re: 'Multiple comparisons and related issues in the interpretation of epidemiologic data.'" *Am. J. Epidemiol.* **147** (1997): 801–6; Goodman, S. N. "Multiple comparisons explained." *Am. J. Epidemiol.* **147** (1997): 807–12; Savitz, D. A. and Olshan, A. F. "Describing data requires no adjustment for multiple comparisons: A reply from Savitz and Olshan." *Am. J. Epidemiol.* **147** (1997): 813–14; Thompson, J. R. "A response to 'Describing data requires no adjustment for multiple comparisons.'" *Am. J. Epidemiol.* **147** (1997): 815.

Delving deeper: Checking the underlying assumptions of the analysis

9.1 How do I know if the assumptions of my multivariable model are met?

In the last chapter, I covered how to assess how well your model fit your data based on those parameters that are typically output by standard computer software packages. In this chapter, we are going to delve deeper to check the underlying assumptions of the models and to determine strategies for improving the fit of models. **Reader beware: keep your biostatistician near for this chapter**. Not only are some of the concepts hard, but many of these supplementary procedures require judgment that comes from having done many prior analyses. Also for many of the issues described below there is controversy as to what procedures are best and whether some have value at all.

The content of this chapter is often referred to as regression diagnostics (as in diagnosing problems with regression models). One of the most useful tools for assessing whether there are problems with the model is analysis of residuals, the subject of the next section. In that section I will review how you can use residuals to assess the overall fit of multivariable models. In the subsequent section I will review how to use residuals and other techniques to identify departures from specific assumptions of multivariable models.

9.2 What are residuals? How are they used to assess the fit of models?

Residuals are the difference between the observed and the estimated value. They can be thought of as the error in estimation.

DEFINITION

Residuals are the difference between the observed and the estimated value.

Besides "raw" residuals, there are a number of possible transformations of residuals for different multivariable procedures (Table 9.1). Standardized and studentized residuals are especially helpful with interpreting linear regression models. Pearson residuals and influence tests are used to interpret multiple logistic regression models. Cox–Snell, Martingale, deviance, and Schoenfeld residuals are useful for interpreting proportional hazards analyses. These

Table 9.1. Type of residual with purposes.

Type of residual used	Purposes
Multiple linear regression	
Raw residuals	Fit of model
	Test of normality and equal variance
	Test of linearity
Standardized residuals	Test of normality and equal variance
	Identification of outliers
Studentized residuals	Identification of outliers that are leverage points
Leverage	Identification of outliers that are leverage points
Cook's distance	Identification of outliers with strong influence
Multiple logistic regression	
Raw residuals	Fit of model
Change in chi-squared statistic with exclusion of subjects with particular covariate pattern	Fit of model, identification of influential observations
Change in deviance with exclusion of subjects with particular covariate pattern	Fit of model, identification of influential observations
Standardized Pearson residuals	Outliers
Change in logistic coefficients with exclusion of subjects with particular covariate pattern	Fit of model, identification of influential observations
Proportional hazards analysis	
Cox–Snell residuals	Fit of model
Martingale residuals	Verification of linearity
Deviance residuals	Identification of outliers
Schoenfeld residuals	Verification of proportionality assumption
Poisson analysis	
Standardized residuals	Fit of model, outliers
Standardized deviance residuals	Fit of model, outliers

different residuals are output by standard software programs, as are the plots described below. I will explain each of these different types of residuals in the context of their specific uses.

To use residuals to assess the overall fit of a multiple linear regression or binary logistic regression model, plot the raw residuals on the y-axis and the estimated outcome on the x-axis. In a well-fitting model, the residuals will be close to 0, meaning that the observed and estimated values are close to one another. When the observed is greater than the estimated value the residual is positive; when the observed value is less, the residual is negative.

When the residuals are larger at certain points of the predicted value of the outcome than at other points (e.g., large at extreme values of the outcome and small at intermediate values) it suggests a violation in the assumptions of the model such as non-normal distribution (Section 9.3), nonlinearity (Section 9.4), or a mis-specification of the model [e.g., an important variable omitted). If there are one or two points with extreme residuals it suggests outliers (Section 9.5)

TIP

Investigate covariate patterns that do not fit well.

For logistic regression it is also helpful in assessing the fit of the model to plot either 1) the change in the value of the Pearson chi-square statistic (based on the Pearson residual) on the y-axis versus the estimated probability of the outcome on the x-axis, or 2) the change in the value of the deviance (based on deletion of subjects with a given covariate pattern) on the y-axis versus the estimated probability of the outcome on the x-axis. Points falling at the top right and left corners of the plot (above the two quadratic curves that you will see at the bottom of the plot) indicate covariate patterns that do not fit well.[1] Investigation of these particular covariate patterns may give you insight into why they do not fit the overall model.

For proportional odds and multinomial regression check the fit of the model by creating two or more (depending on whether you have three or more categories of your outcome variable) binary logistic regression models and assess the fit of each of these models.[2]

For proportional hazards analysis, the fit of the model may be assessed using the Cox–Snell residuals, which can range from zero to infinity. A Kaplan–Meier survival curve for the outcome is generated using the Cox–Snell residuals as the time variable. This curve is then compared to a survival function for the outcome with a unit exponential distribution. If the proportional hazards model fits well the curves will be closely aligned.[3]

For Poisson regression, the fit of the model can be assessed by plotting either the standardized residuals or the standardized deviance residuals against the expected rate of the outcome. Very large (positive or negative) residuals indicate covariate patterns that do not fit the model (outliers). In a well-fitting model 95% of the residuals should be between 2 and –2. If you draw a lowess line you would expect that the line would be flat and near zero. If the line

[1] For a detailed review of residuals with logistic regression see: Hosmer, D. W. and Lemeshow, S. *Applied Logistic Regression*. 2nd edn. New York, NY: Wiley, 2000, pp. 167–86.

[2] Hosmer, D. W. and Lemeshow, S. *Applied Logistic Regression*. 2nd edn. New York, NY: Wiley, 2000, pp. 280–7, 305–8.

[3] For a more detailed discussion of this, along with an illustration and an explanation of an alternative way of using the Cox–Snell residuals to test the fit of the proportional hazards analysis, see: Dupont, W. D. *Statistical Modeling for Biomedical Researchers: A Simple Introduction to the Analysis of Complex Data*. Cambridge: Cambridge University Press, 2002, pp. 239–41.

deviates substantially at certain estimated rates of outcome, it suggests that the model does not fit well at those points.[4]

It is important to understand that residual analysis is more art than science. You may get alarming patterns of residuals even though your data fit the assumptions of your model. For example, with logistic regression you may get residuals that appear disturbing when you have strong dichotomous independent variables (rather than interval-independent variables) even if your model is sound. It is also possible for your residuals to look fine, and yet the assumptions of your model have been violated. Small samples are especially likely to yield messy residuals. With large samples, multivariable models are sufficiently robust that departures from the assumptions of the model seen on residual analysis may not cause significant problems.

> Residual analysis is more art than science.

9.3 How do I test the normal distribution and equal variance assumptions of a multiple linear regression model?

Multiple linear regression assumes normal distribution and equal variance around the mean (Section 3.2.C).

To test whether your outcome has a normal distribution and equal variance around the mean for any value(s) of the independent variable(s), plot the raw residuals against each of the independent variables and the estimated outcome variable. When these assumptions are met the residuals should be close to zero and the spread of values should be equal both above and below zero. If, instead, the residuals are far from zero and there is not an equal spread of values above and below zero, the assumptions of normal distribution and equal variance are not met.[5]

A better method of detecting departures from the normality assumption is to construct a normal probability plot of the standardized residuals. The standardized residuals are simply the residuals divided by the standard deviation of the residuals. A normal probability plot is a plot of the cumulative frequency of the distribution of the residuals versus the residuals on a normal probability graph scale. If the assumption of normality is correct, the plot should be a straight line. A curve indicates that the normality assumption is not true. Points far from the line are outliers (Section 9.5).

> **TIP**
>
> Use normal probability plots to detect departures from the assumptions of normality.

---

[4] For a good example of this type of plot, as well as a discussion of residuals with Poisson analysis see: Dupont, W. D. *Statistical Modeling for Biomedical Researchers: A Simple Introduction to the Analysis of Complex Data.* Cambridge: Cambridge University Press, 2002, pp. 325–6.

[5] For a detailed description of analysis of residuals including numerous graphs see: Glantz, S. A. and Slinker, B. K. *Primer of Applied Regression and Analysis of Variance.* New York, NY: McGraw-Hill, 1990, pp. 110–80.

If your plots do not fit the assumptions of normality and equal variance, don't give up. Look back in the section on transforming variables (Section 3.2.C). It may be that by transforming one of your independent or dependent variables you will achieve a better model. Also, if your sample size is greater than 100, you can assume that the assumption of normal distribution is met for your independent variables (Section 3.2.C).

9.4 How do I test the linearity assumption of a multivariable model?

Residuals can also be used to test the linearity assumption of interval-independent variables entered into a multivariable model. To test whether your interval-independent variables fit a linear relationship with outcome in a linear or binary logistic regression multivariable model, plot your raw residuals against each of your independent variables and the estimated value of the outcome variable. If the relationship is linear, the points will be symmetric above and below a straight line, with roughly equal spread along the line. In contrast, if residuals are particularly large at very high and/or low levels of one of the independent variables or of the outcome variable, it suggests that there may be a departure from linearity.[6]

> **TIP**
>
> Use Martingale residuals to assess the linearity of interval variables with proportional hazards analysis.

In the case of proportional hazards analysis, linearity of interval variables can be assessed using Martingale residuals, which are a linear transformation of Cox–Snell residuals; they range from negative infinity to 1.[7] The Martingale residuals (y-axis) are plotted against the interval predictor (x-axis). The shape of the smoothed curve will indicate whether the relationship is linear or some other shape.[8] This information can help you to determine whether it is necessary to transform your interval variable to satisfy the linearity assumption.

Another method of assessing the linear assumption of interval variables is to create multiple dichotomous variables of equal intervals of your variable. This technique is very flexible and can be used with multiple logistic regression (binary, proportional odds, and multinomial), Poisson regression (including negative binomial regression), and proportional hazards regression; I explained this technique in Section 4.3.C. For multivariable analysis

[6] For a detailed description of analysis of residuals including numerous graphs see: Glantz, S. A. and Slinker, B. K. *Primer of Applied Regression and Analysis of Variance*. 2nd edn. New York, NY: McGraw-Hill, 2001, pp. 113–80.

[7] For a great explanation of the different types of residuals with proportional hazards analysis see: Gillespie, B. "Checking assumptions in the Cox proportional hazards regression model",Center for Statistical Consultation and Research, University of Michigan, 2006, available at: www.lexjansen.com/mwsug/2006/Statistics_DataAnalysis/SD08.pdf.

[8] Hosmer, D. W. and Lemeshow, S. *Applied Logistic Regression*. 2nd edn. New York, NY: Wiley, 2000, pp. 480–2.

you will be using the technique to assess whether your independent variable fits the linearity assumption after adjustment for other independent variables. If the numeric difference between the coefficients of each successive group is approximately equal, this is consistent with a linear gradient.

Finally, some researchers will assess whether an interval variable has a linear gradient by substituting a transformed version of the variable for the variable itself. Commonly, logarithmic and quadratic transformations are tested. If the coefficient for that variable increases and the fit of the model improves with the transformation, this would suggest that the variable more closely fits a logarithmic or quadratic gradient.

9.5 What are outliers and how do I detect them in a multivariable model?

Outliers are points that do not follow the pattern of the other points. For example, Figure 9.1 shows a linear relationship with higher values of the independent variable associated with higher values of the outcome. While most of the points conform to this linear relationship, two points (A and B) do not fit this relationship. Point A has a much higher value for outcome than you would expect given the intermediate value on the independent variable. Point B has a much lower value of outcome than you would expect given the high value of the independent variable.

Although you can gain some insight from the raw residuals, it is easier to detect outliers using standardized residuals, studentized residuals, leverage, and Cook's distance.

Standardized residuals are residuals divided by the standard deviation of the residuals. Because raw residuals depend on the scale of the dependent variable, we cannot set any uniform rules of thumb of what is a large raw residual. However, by standardizing them, we eliminate the units, and can create guidelines for what is a large residual.

Standardized residuals help pinpoint outliers. Standardized residuals larger than two are the extreme 5 percent of values, whereas those larger than three are the extreme 1 percent of values.

Studentized residuals adjust for how far each individual value is from the center of the line. The result is that two points an equal distance from the line will have different studentized residuals: The studentized residual will be larger for the value at the extremes of the line than the value at the center. This is because values at the extremes can exert greater leverage: they can more easily tilt the line. Think of a seesaw, with the center point as the fulcrum and the extreme points as the ends of the plank. Exerting pressure on the end will

> **TIP**
>
> To detect outliers use standardized residuals, studentized residuals, leverage, and Cook's distance.

> **TIP**
>
> Standardized residuals greater than three represent the extreme 1 percent of values.

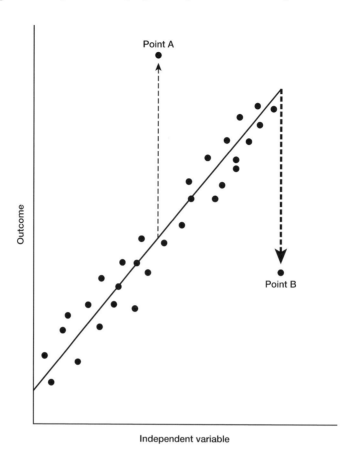

Figure 9.1

Linear relationship between an independent variable and outcome with two outliers (point A and point B). The thicker dotted line pointing to B illustrates the greater leverage of point B compared to point A.

cause the entire plank to change slope. Such points are referred to as leverage points. With studentized residuals, leverage points will get a larger residual than an outlier whose value is close to the center of the line. So in Figure 9.1 point B will have a larger studentized residual than point A even though these points are the same distance from the line. I have used a thicker dotted line in Figure 9.1 to point to B to illustrate the greater leverage of point B compared to point A. As with standardized residuals, studentized residuals of greater than 2–3 suggest problems.

The measure leverage quantifies the leverage of individual points on the line. Ideally, all your observations should have leverage measures less than two times the expected value. The expected value is: (the number of variables

> **TIP**
>
> Outliers at the extremes of the value of the independent value exert greater leverage than those closer to the midpoint.

plus one) divided by the sample size. Leverage values higher than: (two multiplied by the number of variables plus two) divided by the sample size warrant consideration.

Influence refers to how removing an observation changes the estimate of coefficients. Influence is affected by both whether an observation is an outlier and the leverage of that observation. Observations that are outliers and have a large leverage will be influential. Cook's distance assesses how influential an individual point is to the overall model. It is equal to the change in the regression coefficients if the observation was deleted. Cook's distance of greater than four divided by the sample size is cause for concern.

For multivariable (binary) logistic regression, standardized Pearson residuals greater than 2.0 deserve further concern. A plot of the standardized Pearson residuals versus the estimated outcome will show you whether cases are particularly likely to be outliers at particular probabilities of outcome. Remember though with logistic regression we are speaking of covariate patterns (therefore likely multiple cases) rather than a single observation as in multiple linear regression.

For multiple logistic regression there are three methods for identifying influential covariate patterns. All three assess how the model changes when particular covariate patterns are deleted. The three methods are:

1) change in chi-squared statistic
2) change in the deviance
3) change in the regression coefficients.[9]

If you plot each of these changes (y-axis) against the estimated probability of outcome, you may see points that have a particularly strong influence on the result. It is also possible to plot the change in the chi-squared statistic (y-axis) versus the estimated probability of outcome with the size of the circle of the covariate pattern equal to the influence diagnostic parameter. The largest circles will indicate the patterns with the greatest influence.[10]

DEFINITION

Influence refers to how removing an observation changes the estimate of the coefficients of a model.

Cook's distance of greater than four divided by the sample size is cause for concern.

Observations that are outliers and have a large leverage will be influential.

---

[9] This statistic may be referred to as DfBeta or dbeta when only a case is dropped rather than dropping all cases with a particular covariate pattern. In general with logistic regression it makes more sense to drop all cases with a particular covariate pattern when trying to figure out observations that have particular influence on the results.

[10] For a picture of such a curve see: Hosmer, D. W. and Lemeshow, S. *Applied Logistic Regression*. 2nd edn. New York, NY: Wiley, 2000, p. 180.

Outliers can be detected in proportional hazards analysis using deviance residuals. Deviance residuals are a transformation of Martingale residuals which gives them a symmetric distribution around zero. Positive observations have a shorter survival time than expected and negative observations have a longer survival time than expected.[11] If you plot the deviance residual against the subject identification number you will easily see those cases with a particularly high or low residual.

Covariate patterns that are outliers can be detected in Poisson regression with standardized residuals or with standardized deviance residuals.

9.6 What should I do when I detect outliers?

Let's say that your analysis of residuals suggests you have certain extreme values. What do you do? First, check to make sure there is no error in the recording of this data point. You may think that this is an unnecessary step if you have already reviewed your univariate results for extreme values. But review of outliers from multivariable analysis complements the univariate analysis. For example, residual analysis of a multivariable model may detect an obese diabetic with a heavy fat consumption whose cholesterol is abnormally low (140 mg/dl). This may result in your discovering a data-entry error: The value was really 410 mg/dl. Since a cholesterol level of 140 mg/dl is not an extreme value you would not have noticed a problem in the univariate analysis.

But what if you verify from the original data that this subject's value really is 140 mg/dl? Do you delete it from the data set? No. If you were performing a laboratory experiment, and had a residual value that did not fit your analysis, you might want to repeat the experiment. But in clinical trials this is rarely an option. While it may be tempting to delete such values from the study (especially if they are preventing you from getting the answer you were hoping for) this is rarely justified. Just because certain subjects are outliers, it doesn't mean their values are wrong. In fact, it is "normal" to have a few extreme values.

However, if your residuals indicate leverage points, you may want to consider removing them from the analysis, repeating the analysis, and seeing whether your findings hold. If deletion of a couple of observations changes your entire analysis, the analysis may not be valid. In general, the larger your data set is, the less likely it is that your results will be heavily influenced by

---

[11] Gharibvand, L. A step-by-step guide to survival analysis. University of California, Riverside. http://www.wuss.org/proceedings08/08WUSS%20Proceedings/papers/tut/tut08.pdf

one or two points. Therefore, the need to closely examine the residuals of all of your points becomes less important.

When the residuals represent covariate patterns, outliers may represent more than one or two cases, and omitting them may be an unsatisfactory resolution. Therefore, it is more sensible to think of outlying covariate patterns as cases for which the model is not very good at predicting outcome. They deserve further investigation, but not necessarily omission.

9.7 What is the additive assumption and how do I assess whether my multiple independent variables fit this assumption?

All the multivariable models discussed in this book assume that your multiple independent variables have an additive effect on the outcome. Understanding what it means that these multivariable models are additive is complicated because the different models estimate different outcomes. For example, with multiple linear regression the sum of the individual variables estimates the change in the mean value of the outcome. With logistic regression, the sum of the individual independent variables estimates the logit of the outcome. With proportional hazards analysis, the sum of the independent variables estimates the logarithm of the relative hazard. With Poisson regression, the sum of the independent variables estimates the logarithm of the outcome.

A consequence of the additive assumption is that the odds ratios, relative hazards, or relative risks from logistic, proportional hazards, and Poisson regression models (respectively) have a multiplicative rather than an additive, effect on outcome. Statisticians refer to this with the somewhat confusing term of "additive on a multiplicative scale." Although I didn't refer to it as the additive assumption, we have dealt with this concept in the discussion of interactions (Sections 1.4, 7.3, and 8.4). Interactions are present when the variables are not additive but rather something greater or less than additive.

TIP

The effect of multiple variables on the odds ratio or the relative hazard or the relative risk is multiplicative.

If you look back at the discussion on the interaction of gender and ST elevations shown in Section 1.4, you see that I multiplied the odds ratios to show the meaning of the interaction. Specifically, in Table 1.7, the odds ratio for male gender was 1.6 and the odds ratio for ST elevations was 8.1. Since the model is "additive on a multiplicative scale" the odds ratio associated with being male and having ST elevations should be the product of the two or 13.0 $(1.6 \times 8.1 = 13.0)$.

But the risk of heart attack for men with ST elevations was not 13 times the risk for women without ST elevations. How do we know this? Because the product term was statistically significant. To find out the true risk for men with ST elevations, you need to include the interaction term, which had an odds ratio of 0.6. When you include the product term you learn that the risk for men with ST elevations is less than 13.0; it is actually only 7.8 (1.6 × 8.1 × 0.6 = 7.8). After reading Section 8.3B, you would have known that the over-all risk was lower just from the negative sign of the coefficient of the product term.

What does all this mean? Clinically, as discussed in Section 1.4, it means that the difference in the likelihood of heart attacks between men and women vanishes in the presence of ST elevations. (The risk for women with ST eleva-tions is 8.1 (1.0 × 8.1 × 1.0 = 8.1), essentially identical to the risk of 7.8 in men with ST elevations (1.6 × 8.1 × 0.6 = 7.8). In terms of your model, this means that in the absence of including an interaction term for gender and ST eleva-tions, your model would have been mis-specified because the additive assump-tion would not have been fulfilled.

You may be asking yourself, why does the model without interaction terms estimate that men with ST elevations have a significantly higher risk of heart attack than women with ST elevations, if the risk for these two groups is simi-lar? To understand why, remember that each variable (e.g., gender, ST eleva-tions) has only one coefficient. Therefore, the best coefficient for the sample as a whole may not be best for every subgroup of subjects as defined by the independent variables. In other words, just because men have a greater risk of heart attack than women and persons with ST elevations have a greater risk than persons without ST elevations does not mean that men with ST eleva-tions have a greater risk than women with ST elevations. This illustrates how models without product terms can be wrong for particular subsets of subjects. Product terms solve this problem by having another variable that can improve the fit of the model for particular subgroups of subjects.

Assessing whether your variables fulfill the additive assumption becomes especially complicated when you realize that in most analyses there are a large number of possible interaction terms. For example there are forty-five pos-sible two-way interactions between just ten independent variables. And there is nothing to prevent interactions from being three-way (e.g., male × ST eleva-tions × prior heart attack). Short of trying all possible product terms, there is no way to know for certain if your data contain an important interaction.

One clue indicating that you may need an interaction term is that a variable that you thought, based on clinical grounds, would have an important effect on an outcome variable did not. Could it be that the variable is important only under certain conditions? Other clues may come from your analysis of how well your data fit the assumptions of your model. For example, if the standard-ized residuals do not form a straight line on the normal probability plot or if

TIP

The best coefficient for the sample as a whole may not be best for every subgroup of subjects.

your logistic regression residuals are particularly large, the reason may be that you have an interaction.

Besides the fact that interactions are difficult to detect there are other problems. Some statistically significant interactions are very difficult to interpret clinically. In addition, if you test a large number of interactions, it is likely that at least one of them will be statistically significant. Does that mean that this is an important interaction?

In this regard, testing for interaction is similar to performing subgroup analysis. Let's say that a study finds that a new drug is no better than placebo in the sample as a whole. However, when the investigators looked within ten subgroups, they found one group (e.g., hypertensive women with diabetes) for whom the drug worked. Would you conclude that the drug works for hypertensive women with diabetes?

In general, unless there is some reason to believe that the drug should work only in hypertensive women with diabetes, and the authors had therefore planned this subgroup analysis, one would conclude that the drug does not work and the finding was chance. That is, in some subgroups, the drug worked better than placebo. In other subgroups, the drug worked worse than placebo. Overall, there was no effect. The same issue exists if you test ten product terms. If the main effect is null, and nine of the product terms are insignificant, and one of them is significant, do you conclude that overall the drug works in that special condition? Probably not.

Because of these problems, many clinical researchers do not test for interactions at all. In contrast, it is common in the epidemiologic literature to evaluate all possible two-way interactions. The methodological justification is that if a product term is significant, it is improving the statistical quality of the model. However, this strategy is not usually pursued in the medical literature because of the difficulty of making clinical sense out of product terms.

My own preference is to test only for those interactions that are theoretically important. That is the strategy that was pursued in the study described above of the impact of gender on heart attack risk. The researchers evaluated all possible interactions involving gender because it was known that the variables associated with heart attack are different in men and women and because this was the focus of their study. But they did not assess all possible interactions in their data set (e.g., age × race).

Whatever strategy you employ for assessing interactions, it is important to tell your reader whether and how you have tested for interactions. Depending on what strategy you have chosen, you can tell your reader that you:

- tested all primary (second-degree) interactions, or
- tested specific interactions (and detail them), or
- chose not to test any interactions

9.8 How do I test the proportional odds assumption?

You will remember from Section 3.4 that proportional odds regression assumes that the coefficients for the independent variables would be the same regardless of the cut-point of the ordinal variable. To assess whether this assumption is met use the score test. When it is nonsignificant you can assume that the odds ratios are constant across the different cut-points of the outcome variable. Unfortunately, the test may be too sensitive when the sample size is large with the result that you may get a statistically significant score test even if the odds are not that different with the different cut-offs. Therefore, if you have a significant score test, a good first step is to create separate logistic models for each of the possible cut-offs of the outcome variable.[12] Each logistic regression will yield an odds ratio and a confidence interval for each independent variable. You can then compare the odds ratios and their respective confidence intervals at the different cut-offs to each other and to the cumulative odds ratio from the proportional odds regression to determine whether the odds ratios really are different.

9.9 How do I test the proportionality assumption?

Remember from Section 3.9 that for proportional hazards analysis to be valid the proportionality assumption must be true. The assumption is that the hazards for persons with different covariate patterns are constant over time. I illustrated a violation of the proportionality assumption in Figure 3.9. In this figure, we see the two Kaplan–Meier survival curves crossing, because the risk of death is not constant between the two arms of the study.

There are more sophisticated methods for assessing whether the proportional hazards assumption is met. Four commonly used methods are: log-minus-log survival plots, Schoenfeld's partial residuals, dividing time into discrete intervals, and time-dependent covariates.[13] There is no consensus on which of these techniques is best and, appropriately, many investigators will perform more than one test.

[12] Scott, S.C., Goldberg, M.S., and Mayo, N.E. "Statistical assessment of ordinal outcomes in comparative studies." *J. Clin. Epidemiol.* **50** (1997): 45–55.

[13] There is a fifth technique, the Kolmogorov-type supremum test that is increasingly appearing in the literature. However, because the methods are too complicated for this book and because many biostatisticians regard it as an experimental test, I don't discuss it further here; readers who want to know more should see: Lin, D.Y., Wei, L.J., Ying, Z. "Checking the Cox model with cumulative sums of Martingale-based residuals." *Biometrika* **80** (1993): 557–72, available at: http://www.lexjansen.com/mwsug/2006/Statistics_DataAnalysis/SD08.pdf.

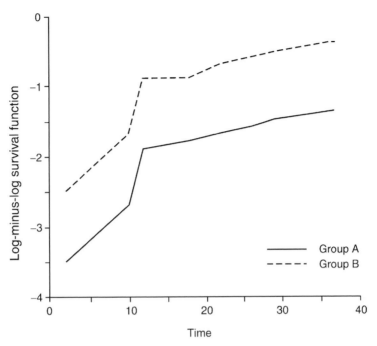

Figure 9.2   Log-minus-log survival plot showing a constant difference between group A (solid line) and group B (broken line). Reprinted with permission from Katz, M.H. and Hauck, W.W. "Proportional hazards (Cox) regression." *J. Gen. Intern. Med.* **8** (1993): 702–11.

9.9.A log-minus-log survival plot

A log-minus-log survival plot is drawn in Figure 9.2. If there is a constant (vertical) difference between the two curves then you know that the hazards of subjects with different values on a particular independent variable are proportional over time. If however, the curves cross, or are much closer together at some points in time and much further apart at other points in time, then the assumption is not true. The curves do not have to be perfectly equidistant. Especially at the ends of the curves, where there tend to be fewer observations, there may be some coming together or greater splitting of the curves.

A nice feature of log-minus-log survival curves is that they illustrate that proportional hazards analysis makes no assumption about the absolute risks (the lines change direction and slope). Proportional hazards analysis only assumes that as the hazards change, the distance between the two curves stays about the same.

9.9.B Schoenfeld's residuals

The proportionality assumption can also be tested using Schoenfeld partial residuals. A plot is drawn of the scaled Schoenfeld's residuals (y-axis) versus a transformation of time (x-axis) for each covariate.[14] If the proportional hazards assumption is met the smoothed line should be approximately horizontal. Some statistical programs (e.g., cox.zph procedure in S-plus) will calculate a chi-squared and P value for each variable, representing the correlation between the scaled Schoenfeld's residuals and transformed time. If the P value is significant then the variable does not fulfill the proportionality assumption.

9.9.C. Divide time into discrete intervals

An intuitively easy way to verify the proportional hazards assumption is to divide the time interval into discrete parts. For example, Liou and colleagues studied the effect of lung transplantation on survival in children with cystic fibrosis.[15] Children had been placed on the waiting list for transplantation over a relatively long period of time. To determine whether the relative hazards of death varied over time for the different independent variables, the investigators divided the study patients by year into two approximately equal-sized groups: those placed on the waiting list between 1992–1998 and those placed on the waiting list between 1999–2002. They then ran two proportional hazards models – one for each sample. Had there been a departure from the proportionality assumption, the relative hazards for the independent variables from the two models would have been different. The authors found that the relative hazards in the two models were similar, thereby supporting the proportionality assumption.

9.9.D. Time-dependent covariates

Another way of testing the proportionality assumption is to add interaction terms to the proportional hazards model that allow the relative hazard to vary

---

[14] For more on how to use Schoenfeld's residuals to check the proportionality assumption see:Fox, J. Cox. Proportional-hazards regression for survival data: Appendix to an R and S-Plus Companion to Applied Regression. February 2002. http://cran.r-project.org/doc/contrib/Fox-Companion/appendix-cox-regression.pdf; Harrell, F.E. *Regression Modeling Strategies: With Application to Linear Models, Logistic Regression, and Survival Analysis*. New York: Springer, 2001, pp. 486–7.

[15] Liou, T.G., Adler, F.R., Cox, D.R., Cahill, B.C. "Lung transplantation and survival in children with cystic fibrosis." *N. Engl. J. Med.* **357** (2007): 2143–52.

over time. The interaction terms are called time-dependent covariates (Section 13.1); they require special coding, which varies with different statistical packages. They can be created so that the logarithm of the relative hazards is allowed to vary linearly with time or with the logarithm of time. When the proportionality assumption is valid, the interaction term will have a hazard ratio near 1.0 (no effect) and will not be statistically significant. If the odds ratio is significantly different from 1.0 it means that the effect of the independent variable does vary over time (the proportionality assumption is not met).

The advantage of time-dependent covariates is that you can create more than one such term and assess simultaneously whether the proportionality assumption is met for multiple independent variables. However, if your sample size is small, you may not be able to enter interaction terms for all variables in the model simultaneously (there may be too many variables for the sample size). In that case, you can add each product term individually to your other variables to see if the product term is significant with adjustment for the other variables in the model. A potential disadvantage of time-dependent covariates is that, if your sample is really large, time interaction terms may be too sensitive. You may get statistically significant terms even though the graphical representation does not show a major departure from the proportionality assumption.

9.10 What if the proportionality assumption does not hold for my data?

You have a few choices (besides abandoning your research career!). You can divide your observation period such that within any one period the odds are proportional. If you do this, you will have two or more proportional hazards analyses. The factors associated with outcome would differ for the two periods (e.g., diabetics will have a higher risk in the model estimating heart attack during the first three months and a lower risk in the model estimating heart attack in the second three-month period).

A second strategy is to perform a stratified proportional hazards analysis. The sample is stratified by the variable that does not fit the proportionality assumption. Each stratum has its own baseline hazard. Therefore each stratum has a component that can vary over time differently from the other strata. The limitations of this strategy are the limitations of any stratified analysis. You cannot assess the effect of the stratification variable on your outcome. Also, stratification is cumbersome if you have more than one or two variables that do not fit the proportionality assumption.

A third strategy is to switch your analysis to logistic regression. Because time is not taken into account in logistic regression models, the risks do not have to be proportional over time. The researchers assessing the factors associated with survival with AIDS in New York City (Section 7.5) switched their model from proportional hazards analysis to logistic analysis after they discovered the proportionality assumption "was seriously violated and could not be remedied through stratification." They created a dichotomous outcome variable: survival for 15 months or longer (yes/no). They found several variables that were associated with survival at 15 months. Although this solution avoided violating the proportionality assumption, one problem is that their results may have been dependent on the cut-off they chose for their outcome. In other words, they may have found different factors associated with survival if they had chosen a cut-off of 6 or 24 months. This is especially problematic because the important research question is: What is associated with survival? Not: What is associated with survival at 15 months? Also, any subjects who were lost to follow-up prior to 15 months would have to be excluded from the analysis. Nevertheless, the researchers deserve credit for verifying the proportionality assumption and adapting their analysis; many authors do not report if and how they assessed the proportionality assumption.[16]

> **TIP**
>
> You can account for the lack of proportionality in a model by allowing the relative hazard to vary by period.

A fourth, and probably the best, strategy is to account for the lack of proportionality in the hazards. In other words, construct your model such that the relative hazard varies by period, taking on one value in the first X time units, another value in the next Y time units, and so on. This approach is analogous to transforming an interval-independent variable (in this case time) into a categorical variable.

For example, my colleagues and I were performing an analysis of the impact of socioeconomic status on survival with AIDS.[17] We assessed the proportionality assumption using log-minus-log survival curves. Most of the curves looked fine. But one of the covariates, an initial AIDS diagnosis of cryptosporidiosis, looked suspicious for violating the proportionality assumption. Because we were not sure, we tested the hypothesis. Instead of the single variable cryptosporidiosis (yes/no), we created two covariates: cryptosporidiosis in the first period of study time (yes/no) and cryptosporidiosis in the second period of study time (yes/no). The cut-off for the time period was chosen based on the log-minus-log survival plot (the point where it seemed the relative hazard changed).

Using proportional hazards analysis we tested the hypothesis that the two variables were significantly different from one another. The P value was only

---

[16] Katz, M. H. and Hauck, W. W. "Proportional hazards (Cox) regression." *J. Gen. Intern. Med.* **8** (1993): 702–11; Concato, J., Feinstein, A. R., and Holford, T. R. "The risk of determining risk with multivariable models." *Ann. Intern. Med.* **118** (1993): 201–10.

[17] Katz, M. H., Hsu, L., Lingo, M., *et al.* "Impact of socioeconomic status on survival with AIDS." *Am. J. Epidemiol.* **148** (1998): 282–91.

marginally significant (0.07). Although this was above the conventional cut-off of P value < 0.05, P values less than < 0.20 can indicate important changes in risk over time. In case this potential departure of the proportionality assumption had an important effect on our overall model, we included these two time-period variables, instead of the one covariate. By having the two covariates in the model, we were no longer violating the proportionality assumption. Because these types of models are complex to set up, it would be best to consult with a biostatistician for help.

No matter what strategy you choose for your analysis, report to the reader how you assessed the assumption and whether it held. If it did not hold, don't feel discouraged. You have learned something, potentially important, about how the risk of your outcome changes over time under certain conditions.

10

Propensity scores

10.1 What are propensity scores? Why are they used?

DEFINITION

Propensity scores
are the likelihood of
a subject being in a
particular treatment
group, conditional on
that subject's values
on those independent
variables thought
to influence group
membership.

Propensity scores are calculations of the likelihood of a subject being in a particular treatment group, conditional on that subject's values on those independent variables thought to influence group membership.[1] They are used to statistically adjust for differences between nonrandomized groups, typically for studies comparing different treatments.[2]

To calculate a propensity score, you first identify the variables that influence treatment group membership, including demographics, disease severity, and characteristics of the treatment system (e.g., physician specialty, hospital, etc.). These variables are entered into a model (typically logistic) estimating the likelihood of treatment group membership. This model yields a score for each subject; the score is the estimated likelihood of being in one group versus the other, conditional on a weighted score of that subject's values on the set of independent variables used to create the propensity score.

To create a propensity
score enter the
variables that influence
treatment group
assignment into a
logistic regression
model estimating
treatment group
membership.

Once calculated there are different ways you can use propensity scores. You can include each subject's propensity score in your multivariable model as an independent variable. Or you can use this score to individually match subjects with different treatment assignments but an equal likelihood of being in a particular group and assess the outcome using a matched analysis (Section 11.1). Alternatively you can assess the likelihood of outcome within quintiles of the propensity score. Attentive readers will recognize that these three different methods of using propensity scores correspond to three different methods for adjusting for baseline differences: multivariable modeling, matching, and

---

[1] Rubin, D. B. "Estimating causal effects from large data sets using propensity scores." *Ann. Intern. Med.* **127** (1997): 757–63; D'Agostino, R. B. "Propensity score methods for bias reduction in the comparison of a treatment to a non-randomized control group." *Statist. Med.* **17** (1998): 2265–81.

[2] For a more detailed discussion of propensity scores, along with two other techniques used when comparing nonrandomized groups – instrumental variable analysis and sensitivity analysis – see: Katz, M. H. *Evaluating Clinical and Public Health Interventions: A Practical Guide to Study Design and Statistics.* Cambridge: Cambridge University Press, 2010, pp. 101–27.

A propensity score can be used in three ways: (1) as a covariate in a multivariable model estimating outcome; (2) as a variable on which to match subjects; (3) as a variable on which to stratify subjects. Propensity scores work especially well when outcomes are rare and the proportions of subjects in the treatment groups are relatively equal.

stratification. A fourth strategy, less commonly used, is to use the propensity score to weight the observations in a multivariable analysis.

But, wait you say! If multivariable analysis (along with matching and stratification) can adjust for baseline differences between nonrandomized groups (Section 2.3), why do we need to complicate things further with propensity scores? Why not simply enter the variables used to construct a propensity score into a multivariable model?

The answer is that propensity scores often produce a better adjustment for baseline differences than simply including potential confounders in your multivariable model. This is especially true when outcomes are rare and the proportions of subjects in the treatment groups are relatively equal.[3] With rare outcomes you often will not have a sufficient sample size to include all the potential confounders in your analysis estimating outcome. Omitting important variables may result in an incorrectly specified model. On the other hand, including too many variables in your multivariable model may result in an unreliable model (Section 6.4). But assuming the distribution of subjects between your groups is relatively equal, then you will have a sufficient sample size to use all your prognostic variables to estimate group assignment. When you return to your model estimating outcome you can enter your propensity score as a single variable stand-in for your multiple potential confounders.

Another advantage of propensity scores is that they make no assumption about the relationship between the individual confounders and the outcome. Of course, for the propensity score to be accurate, the relationship of the independent variables to treatment assignment must fit the assumptions of the model you are using.

Propensity scores were important in demonstrating that right-heart catheterization (a procedure used extensively in critically ill patients during the time I was an internal medicine resident) is not a useful procedure, and may be harmful.

Right-heart catheterization involves inserting a monitoring (Swan–Ganz) catheter directly into the right heart. It began to be widely used in the 1970s without any studies proving its efficacy. Many clinicians felt that the readings enabled them to better monitor and treat their patients. Thus, the practice became the standard of care in certain settings, including the intensive care units of the hospitals I trained in. When some studies found higher rates of death in patients who received right-heart catheterization, the validity of the association between right-heart catheterization and death was questioned

[3] Braitman, L. E. and Rosenbaum, P. R. "Rare outcomes, common treatments: Analytic strategies using propensity scores." *Ann. Intern. Med.* **137** (2002): 693–5.

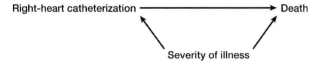

Figure 10.1   Relationships among right-heart catheterization, severity of illness, and death.

because the studies were not randomized. In particular, persons who received right-heart catheterization were known to be sicker than persons who did not receive this procedure. This could have confounded the results of the observation trials, resulting in persons who received right-heart catheterization appearing more likely to die because of the catheterization when they were, in reality, more likely to die because of their underlying disease. This relationship is illustrated in Figure 10.1.

When a randomized controlled trial was launched to definitively answer the question, the study was terminated because physicians were unwilling to randomize their patients. They believed that right-heart catheterization was beneficial; therefore, how could they deny the intervention to their patients?

Since randomization was not an option, Connors and colleagues addressed the effectiveness of right-heart catheterization by prospectively following 5735 critically ill adults cared for in an intensive care unit.[4] Of these, 2184 patients received a right-heart catheterization (38 percent) and 3551 (62 percent) did not. Because the decision of whether or not a patient received a right-heart catheterization was not random, the investigators developed a propensity score to assess the likelihood of each patient receiving a right-heart catheterization. To do this, they had a group of seven specialists in critical care specify the variables they would expect to be related to the decision to use or not use a catheter. They identified over 65 variables to include. These variables were included in a logistic regression analysis estimating the outcome of right-heart catheterization in the first 24 hours of hospitalization. When they adjusted for the propensity score for right-heart catheterization in a proportional hazards analysis, along with additional adjustment for potential confounders, patients managed with a right-heart catheterization had an increased risk of death (OR = 1.21; 95% CI = 1.09 – 1.25) at 30 days.

To strengthen their findings, the investigators also used the propensity scores to perform a matched analysis. Patients managed with and without right-heart catheterizations were matched on the basis of disease category and the propensity score. Patients were matched to the patient with the closest

[4] Connors, A. F., Speroff, T., Dawson, N. V., *et al.* "The effectiveness of right-heart catheterization in the initial care of critically ill patients." *JAMA* **276** (1996): 889–97.

propensity score (within 0.03 on a scale of 0 to 1). This procedure resulted in 1008 pairs (note: not all of the 2184 patients who received a right-heart catheterization could be matched). The likelihood of survival at 30 days was higher for those patients who did not receive right-heart catheterization (67.2) than those who did (62.5) with an odds ratio of 1.24 (95% CI 1.03–1.49).

One ironic aspect of their study is that it created enough uncertainty about the use of right-heart catheterization that a randomized clinical trial became feasible.[5] Published in 2003, seven years after the publication of the study by Connors and colleagues, it showed no benefit for right-heart catheterization among high-risk surgical patients and a higher rate of pulmonary embolism in the catheter group.[6]

> Propensity scores only adjust for measured confounders.

The limitations of propensity scores are similar to the limitations of all forms of multivariable adjustment. Propensity scores can only adjust for measured confounders.

Although you can never adjust for unknown confounders, it is possible to assess how large such a confounder would have to be to affect your results. With the right-heart catheterization study, the investigators used sensitivity analysis to determine how strong a missing confounder would have to be to change the relationship they found from right-heart catheterization being associated with an increased risk of death (OR = 1.21), to right-heart catheterization being associated with a decreased risk of death (OR = 0.80).[7] They found that the missing covariate would have to increase the risk of death six-fold and increase the probability of right-heart catheterization six-fold for the true relative hazard to be 0.80. While this analysis certainly does not prove that such a covariate does not exist, it seems unlikely. This is substantiated by the investigators determining that singly removing the known confounders that have the largest effect on the probability of right-heart catheterization changed the relative hazard of death by only 0.01.

For propensity scores to be effective in adjusting for baseline differences there must be sufficient overlap between the treatment groups on the independent variables you are using to estimate group assignment. One way to assess this is to look at the propensity scores themselves. In the right-heart catheterization study the mean propensity score of patients who received a right-heart catheterization was 0.577 (95 percent confidence interval

[5] Dalen, J.E. and Bone, R.C. "Is it time to pull the pulmonary artery catheter?" *JAMA* **276** (1996): 916–18.
[6] Sandham, J.D., Hull, R.D., Brant, R.F. *et al.* "A randomized, controlled trial of the use of pulmonary-artery catheters in high-risk surgical patients." *N. Engl. J. Med.* **348** (2003): 5–14.
[7] For more on sensitivity analysis see: Rosenbaum, P.R. and Rubin, D.B. "Assessing sensitivity to an unobserved binary covariate in an observational study with binary outcome." *J.R. Stat. Soc.* **45** (1983): 212–18.

0.108–0.943), while the score for those who did not receive a right-heart catheterization was 0.253 (95 percent confidence interval 0.011–0.779).

Test propensity
scores by comparing
the distribution of
independent variables
within quintiles of the
score.

A second important test of whether there is sufficient overlap of the groups is to stratify the groups within quintiles[8] of the propensity score. Then compare the independent variables used to create the scores within the quintiles. You should find similar distributions of the independent variables (e.g., if age is one of the variables used to create a propensity score then the ages of subjects within each of the quintiles should be similar). If not, then there is insufficient overlap between the groups for the propensity score to satisfactorily adjust for baseline differences. This is analogous to adjusting for a confounder using multivariable modeling without a propensity score: to satisfactorily adjust for a confounder there must be sufficient overlap of the groups on the confounder (Section 2.2).

For example, in the right-heart catheterization study, within quintiles of propensity scores there were no differences between those who received and those who did not receive right-heart catheterization on severity of illness, mean blood pressures, heart rate, respiratory rate, pH, PaO_2/FIO_2, $PaCO_2$, disease category, or prognosis.

Despite these limitations propensity scores are the best available method for adjusting for baseline differences in nonrandomized studies of treatments or interventions.

---

[8] The reason for using quintiles is because of an analysis by W. G. Cochran showing that stratification into five or six groups will typically remove 90 percent of the bias present in unadjusted analyses. For a more detailed explanation see: Rubin, D. B. "Estimating causal effects from large data sets using propensity scores." *Ann. Intern. Med.* **127** (1997): 757–63.

Correlated observations

11.1 What circumstances lead to correlated observations?

The multivariable methods that we have discussed thus far assume that each observation (subject) is independent (i.e., the outcomes of different subjects are not correlated). However, it has become increasingly common to study data where the observations are correlated with one another, often referred to as clustered observations or clusters.

As you can see from Table 11.1, a variety of circumstances leads to correlated observations. One common circumstance leading to correlated observations is longitudinal studies, where subjects are observed repeatedly (e.g., baseline and every six months thereafter). Because it is the same subject being observed multiple times, the responses are correlated (i.e., the same subject is more likely to have a similar response each time he or she is observed than a different subject would).

> Repeated observations of subjects in longitudinal studies lead to correlated responses.

Also, when the same subject receives different treatments, as occurs in a crossover study, responses will be correlated because the same person is more likely to respond to different circumstances in a similar way than different individuals receiving different treatments. And the responses of different body parts of the same person (e.g., the right and left eye of Mr. A) will be correlated because the body parts of the same person are more likely to respond similarly than body parts belonging to different persons (e.g., the right eye of Mr. A and the left eye of Mr. B).

Another instance that leads to correlated observations is when subjects are enrolled from established groups or clusters (e.g., families, clinic practices, hospitals, cities) as occurs in randomized and nonrandomized cluster studies. In this case, subjects recruited from the same group are more likely to respond in similar ways than subjects from different groups, leading to correlated outcomes.

Table 11.1 Circumstances leading to and advantages of studying correlated observations.

Circumstance leading to correlated observations	Study design	Advantages of studying correlated observations
Multiple observations of the same subjects at **different times**	Longitudinal study with multiple follow-up assessments	Increases power; strengthens causality
Multiple observations of the same subjects after receiving **different treatments**	Crossover study	Reduces number of subjects who must be recruited; subjects serve as their own control
Multiple observations of **different body parts** of the same subjects	Cross-sectional or longitudinal study	Increases power without recruiting more subjects
Study designs where subjects have been enrolled from randomized or nonrandomized groups (**clusters**) of **related individuals** (e.g., families, doctors' practices, or hospitals)	Clustered randomized or nonrandomized design	Valuable in circumstances where it is easier to enroll subjects by group or when the intervention has an effect on the behavior of the group rather than the individual
Studies where individuals have been randomized at **different centers**	Randomized, multicenter trial	Increases generalizability of the results
Matched study designs where cases and controls have been **individually matched**	Case-control study	Efficient design especially for rare diseases; can be used in circumstances where randomization is not possible

An important instance of correlated observations that is often missed is the multicenter randomized controlled trial.[1] In contrast to the clustered randomized study – where the groups (e.g., hospitals) are randomly chosen, in a randomized multicenter study the individuals are randomized within centers. However, because the responses of subjects within centers are likely to be more closely related to one another than to the responses of subjects within other centers, the observations are correlated.

Finally, when cases have been individually matched to controls, the case is more likely to respond in a similar fashion to the individually matched control than to other controls. Therefore, the analysis must take into account the correlation between cases and their matched control.

---

[1] Localio, A.R., Berlin, J.A., Ten Have, T.R., Kimmel, S.E. "Adjustments for center in multicenter studies: an overview." *Ann. Intern. Med.* **135** (2001): 112–23.

11.2 Should I avoid study designs that lead to correlated observations?

No! Although the analysis of correlated observations is somewhat more complicated than that of independent observations there are a number of important advantages in collecting correlated data (Table 11.1).

First, collecting repeated observations of the same persons can increase the power of your study without increasing the number of subjects. For example, Guskiewicz and colleagues used repeated observations of college football players to assess the effects of recurrent concussion on neurologic function.[2] They followed 2905 players for a total of 4251 player-seasons with an estimated 240, 951 exposures. As you would expect, with multiple observations there are more outcomes. Even so, despite the 240, 951 exposures, only 184 players had a concussion and only 12 had a repeat concussion within the same season.

A second reason for collecting repeated observation of subjects is that it facilitates assessment of time trends. For example, Conter *et al.* studied the effect of maternal smoking during pregnancy.[3] They found that children born to smoking mothers had significantly lower birth weights, but that the rate of growth between 0 and six months of age was greater for babies born to smoking mothers than those born to nonsmoking mothers. The result was that by six months of age the babies of smoking mothers were the same weight as those of nonsmoking mothers. (You have to marvel at the ability of nature to triumph over poison!) Longitudinal observations may also help to establish causality if the effect gets stronger with repeated exposure to the intervention.

Observing the same subject under different conditions can increase the power of your study without increasing your sample size. For example, Paz and colleagues studied the effect of ingestion of ethanol on obstruction of the left ventricular outflow tract in patients with hypertrophic obstructive cardiomyopathy.[4] They performed echocardiography on 36 patients before and after ingestion of ethanol or of placebo. They found that compared to placebo even small amounts of ethanol increased obstruction of the outflow tract – an important finding for patients with hypertrophic obstructive cardiomyopathy who are considering drinking alcohol.

Similarly, if you are studying an outcome in one of the many body parts that occurs in duplicate (e.g., eyes, most joints) or in higher multiples (e.g., teeth, fingers), using all body parts can increase your sample size with the

> **TIP**
>
> Multiple observations of subjects increase the power of a study.

> **TIP**
>
> Use repeated observations of subjects to assess time trends.

---

[2] Guskiewicz, K. M., McCrea, M., Marshall, S. W., *et al.* "Cumulative effects associated with recurrent concussion in collegiate football players." *JAMA* **290** (2003): 2549–55.

[3] Conter, V., Cortinovis, I., Rogari, P., *et al.* "Weight growth in infants born to mothers who smoked during pregnancy." *BMJ* **310** (1995): 768–71.

[4] Paz, R., Jortner, R., Tunick, P. A., *et al.* "The effect of the ingestion of ethanol on obstruction of the left ventricular outflow tract in hypertrophic cardiomyopathy." *N. Engl. J. Med.* **335** (1996): 938–41.

same number of subjects. For example, McAlindon and colleagues studied the relationship of vitamin D to development of osteoarthritis of the knee using data from the Framingham study.[5] Although this cohort consisted of over 5000 subjects, only 556 participants had x-rays of their knees and assessments of their vitamin D intake and serum levels. Therefore, the investigators needed to maximize their statistical power. They did this by looking at both knees. They found that low intake of vitamin D was associated with progression of osteoarthritis of the knee.

A reason you might choose to randomize by group (as in a particular clinic or town) rather than by an individual is that you are interested in interventions that operate on the level of the community, rather than on the level of the individual.[6] For example, you might be interested in studying the effect of the impact of traffic-calming strategies on pedestrian injuries. Also, sometimes it is impossible to randomize individuals within a group because the intervention affects the entire group. For example, Jensen and colleagues randomized nine residential care centers to receive either a multidisciplinary program to reduce falls or standard care.[7] Because the intervention included many center-wide changes such as removing environmental hazards, staff education, and improving transfer techniques, everyone in the center would potentially benefit from the changes. Adjusting their analysis for clustering by center, the investigators found that residents who lived in an intervention center had fewer falls than residents in the centers that did not receive the intervention (OR = 0.49; 95% CI 0.37–0.65).

At other times you may be unable to randomize groups, but instead you will recruit subjects from nonrandomized groups. For example, you may be interested in the effect of air quality on asthma rates. You can't randomize subjects to different levels of air quality, nor can you randomize cities to different levels of air quality. However, you can recruit subjects (randomly or nonrandomly – in this case the randomization is to assure generalizability to the population, not to eliminate bias between cities) from different cities with different levels of air quality and compare their rates of hospitalization for asthma. In such cases, you will need to account for the correlation between subjects living in the same cities.

[5] McAlindon, T. E., Felson, D. T., Zhang, Y., *et al.* "Relation of dietary intake and serum levels of vitamin D to progression of osteoarthritis of the knee among participants in the Framingham study." *Ann. Intern. Med.* **125** (1996): 353–9.

[6] Murray, D. M., Varnell, S. P., and Blitstein, J. L. "Design and analysis of group-randomized trials: A review of recent methodological developments." *Am. J. Public Health* **94** (2004): 423–32.

[7] Jensen, J., Lundin-Olsson, L., Nyberg, L., *et al.* "Fall and injury prevention in older people living in residential care facilities: A clustered randomized trial." *Ann. Intern. Med.* **136** (2002): 733–41.

Another advantage of using established groups to collect data is that it can be logistically simpler. For example, Gandhi and colleagues assessed adverse drug events in 661 patients seen by 24 physicians.[8] Because physician practice style would be expected to influence prescribing practices, the investigators needed to adjust for clustering by physicians. However, it would have been a logistic nightmare to review the medical records of 661 patients seen by 661 physicians. At this point you might wonder why not just study 661 patients from the same physician. Then you would not have to adjust for clustering by physician and you would have an easy job with data collection. The problem is that when you collect data from a single practitioner your data are not very generalizable.

Increased generalizability is also the reason that randomized multicenter trials are such a strong study design. By randomizing patients at multiple centers we have greater confidence that the results will apply to a broad group of patients than if we randomize patients at only a single site. However, we must then adjust for the correlation between the subjects at the same centers.

Finally, the reason we conduct individually matched studies is to decrease confounding (the key word here is individually matched; it is not a matched design if you choose controls that as a whole are comparable to the cases). Matching cases and controls on potentially confounding variables will enable you to answer the same question with a smaller sample because you will no longer have to adjust for differences between the cases and the controls on the variables for which you have matched (they are the same for each pair of cases and controls).

11.3 How do I analyze correlated observations?

> Failure to account for nonindependent observations will result in inaccurate standard errors, *P* values, and confidence intervals.

Regardless of why you have correlated data, you will need multivariable methods that adjust for the correlations (Table 11.2).[9] Failure to do so will result in inaccurate standard errors, leading to inaccurate *P* values and confidence intervals.

Although there are major differences in these methods, one commonality is that you will need to have a variable that identifies repeated or related observations. Without such a variable there would be no way for the software to know which observations are repeated or related. In the case of repeated

---

[8] Gandhi, T. K., Weingart, S. N., Borus, J., *et al.* "Adverse drug events in ambulatory care." *N. Engl. J. Med.* **348** (2003): 1556–64.

[9] For a review of bivariate statistics for analyzing correlated observations see: Katz, M. H. *Study Design and Statistical Analysis: A Practical Guide for Clinicians.* Cambridge: Cambridge University Press, 2006, pp. 107–19.

Table 11.2 Methods for studying correlated observations.

Method	Features
Transform into a single measure Change score Slope	May be used with repeated observations of the same subject on an interval outcome. Change scores are useful when there are only two time points. Slopes can accommodate multiple observations, an unequal number of observations per cluster, and unequal time intervals between observations, but can only be used for linear trends.
Generalized estimating equations (also called a marginal model or a population-averaged model)	Models the effect of intervention/exposure within and among clusters. Can model a variety of different relationships between risk factors and outcomes; adjustment widens confidence interval but does not change point estimate. Can accommodate unequal number of observations and unequal time intervals between observations.
Mixed-effects models (also called multilevel models, random effects regression models, random coefficient models, and hierarchical models)	Models the individual-level effect of the intervention/exposure (within cluster effect only). Can model a variety of different relationships between risk factors and outcomes; adjustment affects both the point estimate and the confidence interval. Can accommodate unequal number of observations and unequal time intervals between observations.
Repeated measures analysis of variance	Can only be used with interval outcomes, an equal number of observations per subject and fixed periods between observations.
Conditional logistic regression	May only be used with dichotomous outcomes, an equal number of observations per subject, and fixed periods between observations.
Anderson–Gill counting process for proportional hazards analysis	Adaptation of proportional hazards analysis for repeated outcomes of a time-to-outcome variable.
Marginal approach for proportional hazards analysis	Adaptation of proportional hazards analysis for repeated outcomes of a time-to-outcome variable.

TIP

With correlated observations you need to specify a variable that identifies the observations that are repeated or related.

observations of the same person this variable may be the identification number of the subject. In the case of data from clustered groups, it will be the identification of the group (e.g., the medical practice or the hospital) from which the case was drawn. For individually matched data, you will need a variable identifying each matched set of observations (i.e., the variable could be called match, and the value of the variable for the first pair of matches could be 1, the value of the variable for the second pair of matches could be 2, etc.).

Having created a common identifier, you may next wish to measure the strength of the correlation between observations. At first blush you might think you could do this with the correlation coefficient. But the correlation coefficient measures the correlation between variables not between linked observations. The intraclass correlation tells you how strong the correlation is between linked observations. The larger the coefficient the stronger the correlation of the observations and the greater the impact adjusting for the correlation will have on your results.

> **DEFINITION**
>
> The intraclass correlation tells you how strong the correlation is between linked observations.

The different methods of adjusting for correlated observations are discussed in Sections 11.3.A to 11.3.F.

11.3.A Transform repeated observations into a single measure

One straightforward method of analyzing repeated observations of a subject is to transform the repeated observations into a single measure. This can be done using a change score. A change score is the absolute or relative change of an outcome variable over the study period.

> **DEFINITION**
>
> A *change score* is the absolute or relative change of your outcome variable over the study period.

For example, Penninx and colleagues were interested in assessing whether depression contributes to subsequent functional decline in older persons.[10] They assessed the physical performance of 1286 elders at baseline and then four years later. To determine the absolute change in performance, they subtracted the baseline score from the follow-up score. They then used change in performance as their outcome measure. Because they used a single change score rather than the two correlated observations, they were able to use multiple linear regression, without adjustment for the correlation between observations. They found that older persons who reported depressive symptoms were at higher risk of subsequent physical decline.

Change scores can also be adapted to weigh relative changes more than absolute changes. This is done by dividing the change score by the baseline score. For example, with CD4 lymphocyte counts (an immunologic measure used to assess persons with HIV disease), a 100-cell change in six months would more likely be associated with progression of disease, if it reflected a drop from 200 cells to 100 cells than if it reflected a drop from 1200 cells to 1100 cells. Both result in an absolute change of 100 cells but the relative change of the former is much larger (100/200 = 0.5) than the latter (100/1200 = 0.08).

Change scores will not work when you have more than two observations. However, you can develop a measure of change over the course of the study period. This is usually done by plotting the observations for each case over time and determining the slope for each case. You can then use the slope as

---

[10] Penninx, B. W. J. H., Guralnik, J. M., Ferrucci, L., *et al.* "Depressive symptoms and physical decline in community-dwelling older persons." *JAMA* **279** (1998): 1720–6.

a continuous outcome variable. This works well for variables that increase (or decrease) in a linear fashion over time. Continuing with the example of serial CD4 lymphocyte counts, the slope of the CD4 count is often used by investigators as a measure of the rate of progression of disease over time because these counts decrease in a linear fashion (in the absence of therapy).[11]

Analogous to dividing a change score by the baseline value, you can divide the slope by its intercept. The result will be that changes that occur in subjects with high intercepts will be weighted less than changes that occur at the lower values. This method was used by Riggs and colleagues to evaluate change in bone mineral density in their study of fluoride treatment of osteoporosis.[12]

An advantage of slopes is that they can be performed when you have an unequal number of observations between clusters (e.g., one subject has four observations and a different subject has six observations) or when you have unequal time intervals between observations (e.g., one subject has measurements at 3 months, 6 months and 18 months and a different subject has measurements at 6 months, 12 months and 24 months).

To calculate a slope only two points at any time are needed. However, researchers usually will set a minimum of points needed to have a valid slope. (For example, Phillips and colleagues included only subjects who had at least five measurements of their CD4 count.[11]) If the minimum number of measurements is not available, the case is excluded.

Although the use of change scores or slopes may seem simplistic, it can be a very powerful method of dealing with repeated observations. For example, D'Amico *et al.* used slopes to characterize changes in prostate-specific antigen (PSA) levels (PSA velocity) among patients with prostate cancer.[13] Over a thousand men were followed for an average of five years, with PSA levels measured about every six months. They found that men with a PSA velocity of more than 2.0 ng per milliliter per year were significantly more likely to die from prostate cancer than men who had smaller changes in their serial PSA levels.

A disadvantage of slopes is that they only apply when the outcome changes linearly over time. Any other time trend would yield incorrect results when analyzed by this method. (Any change between two points can be statistically treated as linear.)

[11] Phillips, A. N., Lee, C. A., Elford, J., *et al.* "Serial CD4 lymphocyte counts and development of AIDS." *Lancet* **337** (1991): 389–92.

[12] Riggs, B. L., Hodgson, S. F., O'Fallon, W. M., *et al.* "Effect of fluoride treatment on the fracture rate in postmenopausal women with osteoporosis." *N. Engl. J. Med.* **322** (1990): 802–9.

[13] D'Amico, A. V., Chen M-H., Roehl, K. A., *et al.* "Preoperative PSA velocity and the risk of death from prostate cancer after radical prostatectomy." *N. Engl. J. Med.* **351** (2004): 125–35.

11.3.B Generalized estimating equations

Generalized estimating equations represent an extremely flexible method of adjusting for correlated observations.[14] They can be used to model a variety of different relationships between the risk factors and an outcome including linear, logistic, or logarithmic; generalized estimating equations can be used with interval, dichotomous, ordinal, and categorical outcomes;[15] `they allow for inclusion of independent variables that do not change (fixed variables such as ethnicity) as well as variables that change at each observation (e.g., blood pressure).

> Generalized estimating equations are population-averaged models.

Generalized estimating equations are population-averaged models (also referred to as marginal models). The mean of the dependent variable is modeled as a function of the independent variables, assuming that the variance is a known function of the mean.[16] Generalized estimating equations are classified as unconditional models because they estimate the effect without regard to what cluster the individual is from. Therefore, estimates from generalized estimating equations represent the joint impact of within- and among-cluster effects of the treatment or exposure.[1]

> Generalized estimating equations estimate the effect of treatment or exposure both within and among clusters.

Generalized estimating equations can incorporate different numbers of observations for different clusters (e.g., two observations for one subject and four observations for another subject; 20 subjects from one hospital and 40 subjects from a different hospital). This is a major advantage of this method.

In cases where the different number of observations stems from missing data, you have to distinguish between data that are not missing at random, also referred to as "nonignorable" or "informative" missing data, and data that are missing randomly, also referred to as "ignorable" missing data.[17] Missing data is nonignorable if (1) the occurrence of a missing value can be predicted by a prior value of the outcome (e.g., patients with missing CD4 counts are more likely to have had a low CD4 count prior to the missing value); and/or (2) certain groups of patients are more likely to have a missing value on the

---

[14] For a comprehensive text of generalized linear models see: Hardin, J. W. and Hilbe, J. M. *Generalized Estimating Equations*. Boca Raton, FL: Chapman & Hall, 2003; for more on the original development of the methods see: Zeger, S. L. and Liang, K.-Y. "Longitudinal data analysis using generalized linear models." *Biometrika* **73** (1986): 13–22; Zeger, S. L. and Liang, K.-Y. "Longitudinal data analysis for discrete and continuous outcomes." *Biometrics* **42** (1986): 121–30.

[15] For an ordinal outcome, the model underlying generalized estimating equations would be proportional odds logistic regression. For a good example of how to set up such a model see: Tishler, P. V., Larkin, E. K., Schluchter, M. D., *et al.* "Incidence of sleep-disordered breathing in an urban adult population." *JAMA* **289** (2003): 2230–7.

[16] Murray, D. M., Varnell, S. P., and Blitstein, J. L. "Design and analysis of group-randomized trials: A review of recent methodological developments." *Am. J. Public Health* **94** (2004): 423–32.

[17] In their classic test, Little, R. J. A. and Rubin, D. B. *Statistical Analysis with Missing Data*. New York, NY: John Wiley and Sons, 1987, distinguish three types of missing data: "data missing completely

outcome (e.g., Caucasian women are more likely to have a missing observation for bone density than women of other ethnicities).

To test whether observations are missing randomly assign each subject a value of 0 or 1, depending on whether or not the subject has one or more missing observations on the outcome. Using multivariable logistic regression, test the association between this variable and the independent variables and the prior values of the outcome. If the data are missing randomly, there should be no association between the independent variables and the prior values of the outcome, and whether or not the subject has missing values.

Generalized estimating equations can accommodate missing responses if the data are missing randomly.[18] Some investigators have found that when the outcome variable is continuous (but not when it is dichotomous), generalized estimating equations may also accommodate missing data that are not missing randomly.[19] My view is that when you have a lot of missing data or nonrandom missing data you need to worry that your analysis is biased. On the other hand, small amounts of data, or data that you can empirically show are ignorable, are unlikely to cause problems with generalized estimating equations.

Another advantage of generalized estimating equations is that they can handle unequal intervals between observations.

The effect of generalized estimating equations is to increase the standard errors (and therefore the confidence intervals) of the point estimates as a reflection of the correlation of clustered observations. However, generalized estimating equations do not change the point estimates (e.g., regression coefficients, odds ratios) themselves.

For example, in a study related to the one described at the start of this chapter, McCrea and colleagues used generalized estimating equations to evaluate the effect of concussion on cognitive function among collegiate football players.[20] Injured athletes and uninjured controls were assessed on repeated occasions. Generalized estimating equations were needed to adjust for correlations between repeated observations of the same person. Potential confounders included in the model were baseline neuropsychiatric function, academic year, number of previous concussions, history of learning disability, and collegiate institution. The study found that athletes with concussion exhibited mild

TIP

Evaluate your missing data by using logistic regression to test the association between having missing values and the independent variables and the prior values of your outcome variable.

Generalized estimating equations can handle unequal intervals between observations.

In adjusting for correlated outcomes, generalized estimating equations change the standard errors but not the point estimates.

at random," "data missing at random," and "data not missing at random." However, in practice, most investigators distinguish just two groups: missing at random or not missing at random.

[18] Diggle, P. J., Heagerty, P., Liang, K-Y., and Zeger, S. L. *Analysis of Longitudinal Data* (2nd edn). Oxford: Oxford University Press, 2002, p. 284.

[19] Twisk, J. W. R. *Applied Longitudinal Data Analysis for Epidemiology: A Practical Guide.* Cambridge University Press, 2003, pp. 208–12.

[20] McCrea, M., Guskiewicz, K. M., Marshall, S. W., *et al.* "Acute effects and recovery time following concussion in collegiate football players." *JAMA* **290** (2003): 2556–63.

Table 11.3 Types of working correlation matrices for generalized estimating equations.

Type	Description	When to use
Exchangeable working correlation matrix (also referred to as compound symmetric working correlation).	Assumes that any two observations within a cluster have the same correlation.	Most common choice for analyzing data for nonindependent observations.
M-dependent structure.	Assumes that the correlation of any two measurements an equal distance apart within a cluster are the same.	May use when correlations between repeated observations are known to decrease as the distance between them increases.
First-order autoregressive correlation model (also known as the exponential correlation model).	Assumes that the correlation within a cluster decreases (in an exponential fashion) as the distance between observations increases.	May use when correlations between repeated observations are known to decrease over time (e.g., longitudinal studies).
Independent correlation model.	Assumes that the repeated observations within a cluster are independent (are not correlated).	May be used for studies where the number of observations per cluster is small relative to the number of clusters.
Unstructured correlation model.	Makes no assumption about the correlation of observations within a cluster.	May use when the number of observations within a cluster is small and balanced. Otherwise computationally difficult.

impairment in cognitive processing speed and fluency two and seven days after concussion compared to uninjured controls.

To run a model using generalized estimating equations you will need to specify three things:

(1) a link function
(2) a working correlation matrix
(3) a method for estimating the variance–covariance matrix

The link function is the type of model you are using to fit to your data. Common choices are linear, logit, or log. Each model has a corresponding distribution of the random component (Gaussian [normal], binomial or Poisson, respectively).

The working correlation matrix indicates how the observations of each cluster are related to one another. You have several choices as shown in Table 11.3.

The most common choice for a working correlation matrix for correlated observations is the exchangeable working correlation matrix (also referred to as a compound symmetric working correlation). This structure assumes that

The exchangeable working correlation matrix assumes that any two correlated observations are correlated equally.

any two correlated observations are correlated equally (e.g., the first and third observations of a particular subject have the same correlation as the first and second observations of that subject, but a [possibly] different correlation than that of the observations of a different subject, or the first and third child in a family have the same correlation as the first and second child in that family, but a [possibly] different correlation than two children from a different family).

In some cases the assumption of equal correlations within clusters will not be true. Certain observations may be more highly correlated than others (e.g., observations of the same individual that are close in time are usually more highly correlated than those that are far apart in time; siblings who are close in age may respond more similarly than siblings born far apart). The correlation matrix may be different for different groups of subjects (e.g., the observations of patients from small hospitals may be more highly correlated than the observations of patients at larger hospitals).

The M-dependent structure assumes that the correlations of observations measured an equal distance apart within a cluster are equal. In other words, the correlation of any two measurements six months apart is equal, the correlation of any two measurements a year apart is equal, etc. With the M-dependent structure you can also stipulate that the correlation of measurements that are separated far in time (time equals M) is zero.

The first-order autoregressive working correlation matrix (also known as the exponential correlation model) assumes that the correlation between repeated/related observations within a cluster decreases (in an exponential fashion) as observations are further apart. This is often the case with longitudinal studies.

The independent correlation matrix assumes that the repeated measurements within a cluster are independent. You may wonder why I would even include it among your choices for dealing with correlated outcomes. The reason is that when the number of clusters is large relative to the number of observations per cluster, the impact of the correlation may be small enough to ignore. When using generalized estimating equations with an independent correlation matrix and a normally distributed interval outcome, the procedure is the same as fitting a linear regression model.[21]

As implied by the name, the unstructured working correlation matrix makes no assumption about how the data within a cluster are correlated. This may seem like a major advantage since the true correlation matrix may be unknown. However, when there are many observations and/or a varying

[21] Davis, C.S. *Statistical Methods for the Analysis of Repeated Measurements.* New York, NY: Springer-Verlag, 2003, p. 297.

number of observations, the unstructured working correlation matrix is hard to estimate accurately.

Although the goal is to choose a working correlation structure that fits your data, it turns out that the generalized estimating equation analysis only needs a rough estimate of the true correlation structure to get started; the final parameter estimates are not generally dependent on the accuracy of the choice of working correlation matrix.[22] Therefore you should take into account the computational difficulty of the different working correlation matrices. For this reason, the exchangeable structure, which is computationally easier than the M-dependent, autoregressive or unstructured correlation structure, is often chosen.

The variance–covariance structure is a function of the working correlation and the link function. The two commonly used methods for estimating it are the Huber–White sandwich estimator and a model-based estimate. In general, the Huber–White sandwich estimator is preferred since it makes no assumption about the variance model; because it will produce correct inferences even when the chosen correlation structure is incorrect, the standard errors are said to be robust. Unfortunately, the estimator is biased downward (i.e., the standard errors will not be accurately inflated, resulting in overstating the significance of the results) when the number of clusters is small (< 40).[23] Therefore the model-based estimate is preferred when the number of clusters is small, especially less than 20.[24]

Once you have chosen your link function, a working correlation matrix, and a method for estimating the variance–covariance matrix, you can conduct your analysis. Your output will look similar (i.e., coefficients, standard errors, P values for your different risk factors) to a standard analysis (e.g., linear regression, logistic regression, or Poisson regression) but the standard errors will be adjusted for the correlation within your clusters.

> **TIP**
>
> In most cases you will want to specify an exchangeable working correlation matrix.

> **TIP**
>
> Unless the number of clusters is small, use the Huber–White sandwich estimator.

11.3.C Mixed-effects model

Perhaps the most confusing aspect of mixed-effects models is all the different names that this procedure goes by in the literature: mixed models, random effects regression models, random coefficient models, random-regression

[22] Dupont, W. D. *Statistical Modeling for Biomedical Researchers: A Simple Introduction to the Analysis of Complex Data.* Cambridge: Cambridge University Press, 2002, pp. 356–67.

[23] Murray, D. M., Varnell, S. P., and Blitstein, J. L. "Design and analysis of group-randomized trials: A review of recent methodological developments." *Am. J. Pub. Health* **94** (2004): 423–32.

[24] Horton, N. J. and Lipsitz, S. R. "Review of software to fit generalized estimating equation regression models." *American Statistician* **53** (1999): 160–9.

models, multilevel models, and hierarchical models. Some authors add the word linear to describe them, as in: linear mixed-effects models or hierarchical linear models. The linear is added to distinguish them from nonlinear mixed-effects models, which can also be constructed.

The different names of these models refer to different features of them. Mixed-effects models are referred to as "mixed" because they contain both fixed and random effects. The models assume that individuals deviate randomly from the average (fixed) response. The underlying fixed model may be linear, logistic, or Poisson. Because of the random effect, the slope and intercept of each individual subject may be different.[25]

These models are referred to as "multilevel" or "hierarchical" because they incorporate two or more "levels" of "random" variation where one level is "higher" than the other. For example, 1000 patients (level 1) may be cared for by one of 100 treating physicians (level 2) working in one of ten hospitals (level 3). Observations are correlated (clustered) at each of these levels.

Although you might think from this explanation that you cannot use these models to analyze repeated observations of the same subject, this is not true. Repeated observations (level 1) are clustered at the "higher" level of the subject (level 2). Similarly, observations of two body parts (level 1) of the same subject are clustered at the level of the subject (level 2) as well.

An example of clustered data that does not fit a hierarchical model would be surgical complication rates of physicians who work in multiple different hospitals. Because the physicians do not exclusively work in one hospital, they cannot all be fitted within a higher level. Although multiple-level nonhierarchical mixed-effects models are available, they are computationally difficult and their use is controversial.[26]

In contrast to generalized estimating equations which are unconditional models, mixed-effects models are conditional models. They estimate the individual-level impact of the intervention/exposure conditional on the cluster (within-cluster effect only).

> Models are conditional: they estimate the individual-level impact of the intervention/exposure conditional on the cluster.

As with generalized estimating equations, mixed-effects models can incorporate interval, dichotomous, ordinal, and categorical outcomes, as well as independent variables that are fixed and those that may change value at each observation.

Unlike generalized estimating equations, for which you must specify a correlation structure, mixed-effects models assume that the correlation within

[25] Ker, H.-W., Wardrop, J., and Anderson, C. Applicaton of linear missed-effects models in longitudinal data: A case study. http://www.hiceducation.org/edu_proceedings/hsiang-wei%20ker.pdf.
[26] Panageas, S. S., Schrag, D., Riedel, E., *et al.* "The effect of clustering of outcomes on the association of procedure volume and surgical outcomes." *Ann. Intern. Med.* **139** (2003): 658–65.

the cluster arises from the common random effects of the cluster. It is also possible to specify a variance and correlation structure, and use your data to estimate its parameters.[27]

As is true of generalized estimating equations, mixed-effects models can handle unequal intervals between observations, unequal numbers of observations per cluster, and randomly missing data. Again as with generalized estimating equations, some authors report that mixed-effects models can handle data that are not missing randomly when the outcome is interval (but not when the outcome is dichotomous).[28] However, I would be cautious about using these models if you have a lot of missing data (because you can never be sure if the data are missing randomly), or when you know the data are not missing randomly.

With a dichotomous outcome, the meaning of the coefficients differs between generalized estimating equations and mixed-effects models. With generalized estimating equations, the coefficient is the between-person difference in the log odds of the outcome comparing the effect of the intervention to no intervention (or the effect of being in one group to being in a different group) as if the intervention and the no intervention (or the group assignment) had been performed on two separate individuals. The coefficient in the mixed-effects models is the within-person change in the log odds of the outcome comparing the effect of the intervention to no intervention as if the intervention had been performed on the same individual.[29] Unlike generalized estimating equations, mixed-effects models can change the point estimate of effect as well as the confidence intervals.

Kandel and colleagues used a mixed-effects model to study racial and ethnic differences in cigarette smoking among adolescents.[30] The data were drawn from a representative sample of 90, 118 adolescents. The investigators used a three-level hierarchical model: adolescents (level 1), school (level 2), and state (level 3). Observations of adolescents within the same school would be expected to be correlated because of characteristics particular to each school (e.g., principal, equipment) and observations from schools within the same state would be expected to be correlated because of similar statewide education policies.

[27] Gueorguieva, R. and Krystal, J. H. "Move over ANOVA: Progress in analyzing repeated-measures data and its reflection in papers published in the Archives of General Psychiatry." *Arch. Gen. Psychiatry* **61** (2004): 310–17.

[28] Twisk, J. W. R. *Applied Longitudinal Data Analysis for Epidemiology: A Practical Guide.* Cambridge University Press, 2003, pp. 208–12.

[29] Murray, D. M., Varnell, S. P., and Blitstein, J. L. "Design and analysis of group-randomized trials: A review of recent methodological developments." *Am. J. Public Health* **94** (2004): 423–32.

[30] Kandel, D. B., Kiros, G.-E., Schaffran, C., *et al.* "Racial/ethnic differences in cigarette smoking initiation and progression to daily smoking: A multilevel analysis." *Am. J. Public Health* **94** (2004): 128–35.

A hierarchical structure works because each school is in a particular state and children do not attend more than one school. The study found that transition to daily smoking was significantly higher among white and Hispanic youth than among black youth.

An advantage of mixed-effects models over generalized estimating equations is that they require no minimum sample size for a particular group.[31]

In addition, if your focus is on predicting how the values of individual units (e.g., persons, clinics, hospitals) change rather than the mean of the population, mixed-effects models are a better choice than generalized estimating models.[32] For example, it would be better to use a mixed-effects model for predicting the bone mineral density of a 66-year-old Caucasian woman with a history of smoking and alcohol consumption, and use the generalized estimating model to estimate the impact of age, smoking, and alcohol consumption on average bone marrow density in a sample of community elders.

With interval outcomes the results from generalized estimating equations and mixed-effects models will be similar. Of note, two articles on the same topic (relationship of procedure volume on mortality in cardiac patients) published in the same issue of the same journal used different techniques: Magid and colleagues used generalized estimating equations to adjust for within-hospital clustering and McGrath and colleagues used mixed-effects models to adjust for clustering of physicians.[33]

11.3.D Repeated measures analysis of variance/repeated measures analysis of covariance

Repeated measures analysis of variance is an adaptation of analysis of variance. It is used to compare means of an interval outcome measure (e.g., cholesterol level) when you have two or more groups defined by an experiment or characteristic (e.g., ethnicity). Additional categorical independent variables can be incorporated into repeated measures analysis of variance (e.g., occupation).

Unlike generalized estimating equations and mixed-effects models, repeated measures analysis of variance can only accommodate interval outcome

> **TIP**
> Choose mixed-effects models over generalized estimating equations when you have a small number of clusters or when your focus is predicting outcomes of specific individuals.

> With interval outcomes the results from generalized estimating equations and mixed-effects models will be similar.

> **DEFINITION**
> Repeated measures analysis of variance is used to compare means for two or more groups on repeated observations of an interval variable.

[31] Christiansen, C. L. and Morris, C. N. "Improving the statistical approach to health care provider profiling." *Ann. Intern. Med.* **127** (1997): 764–8.

[32] Diggle, P. J., Heagerty, P., Liang, K.-Y., *et al. Analysis of Longitudinal Data* (2nd edn). Oxford: Oxford University Press, 2002, p. 130; Davis, C. S. *Statistical Methods for the Analysis of Repeated Measurements.* New York, NY: Springer-Verlag, 2003, pp. 294–8.

[33] Magid, D. J., Calonge, B. N., Rumsfeld, J. S., *et al.* "Relation between hospital primary angioplasty volume and mortality for patients with acute MI treated with primary angioplasty vs thrombolytic therapy." *JAMA* **284** (2000): 3131–8; McGrath, P. D., Wennberg, D. E., Dickens, J. D., *et al.* "Relation between operator and hospital volume and outcomes following percutaneous coronary interventions in the era of the coronary stent." *JAMA* **284** (2000): 3139–44.

variables and independent variables that are fixed (i.e., do not change their value during the course of the study).

Another disadvantage of repeated measures analysis of variance is that you must have the same number of observations of each subject and the observations must be made at the same time. This explains why repeated measures analysis of variance and covariance is more likely to be used with small experiments than with larger observational studies. If you have missing data, as is almost always the case with observational data, you must impute the data point, carry the last observation forward or drop the case from the analysis. Any of these strategies, especially the latter two, are likely to bias your analysis.

Although standard repeated measures models require an equal number of observations, repeated measures analysis of variance for an unequal number of observations (referred to as unbalanced designs) exist.[34] However, these methods are complicated and require consultation with a biostatistician. When you have clusters with an unequal number of observations, it is generally better to choose generalized estimating equations or mixed-effects models.

Despite these limitations, repeated measures analysis of variance is a perfectly acceptable method of analyzing small experimental studies with an equal number of observations made at the same point in time in each cluster. For example, Schmidt and colleagues used repeated measures analysis of variance to tease out the cause of premenstrual syndrome.[35] Ten women with premenstrual syndrome were compared to 15 women without the syndrome on their response to leuprolide (a gonadatropin-releasing hormone agonist) or leuprolide plus hormone replacement. The investigators found a significant interaction between treatment group (leuprolide alone or with hormone replacement), diagnosis (women with premenstrual syndrome or not), and week of study. Specifically, women with premenstrual syndrome experienced greater sadness and more anxiety at week three after receiving leuprolide and hormone replacement than after receiving only leuprolide. Also at week three, women with the premenstrual syndrome who received leuprolide plus hormone treatment experienced more sadness and anxiety than women without this syndrome. The findings suggest that women with premenstrual syndrome experience an abnormal response to normal hormonal changes.

Repeated measures analysis of covariance is similar to repeated measures analysis of variance but it allows for incorporation of continuous independent

[34] Jennrich, R. I. and Schluchter, M. D. "Unbalanced repeated-measures models with structured covariance matrices." *Biometrics* **42** (1986): 805–20.

[35] Schmidt, P. J., Nieman, L. K., and Danaceau, M. A. "Differential behavioral effects of gonadal steroids in women with and in those without premenstrual syndrome." *N. Engl. J. Med.* **338** (1998): 209–16.

Table 11.4 Effect of cognitive behavior therapy (treatment group) versus usual therapy (control group) for patients with hypochondriasis.

	Treatment group ($n = 102$) mean (95% CI)	Control group ($n = 85$) mean (95% CI)	P value
Whiteley index baseline	3.58 (3.47–3.68)	3.51 (3.38–3.62)	<0.001
6-month follow-up	2.82 (2.68–2.97)	3.21 (3.05–3.38)	
12-month follow-up	2.65 (2.48–2.81)	3.02 (2.85–3.21)	

Barsky, A. J. and Ahern, D. K. "Cognitive behavior therapy for hypochondriasis: A randomized controlled trial." *JAMA* **291** (2004): 1464–70.

variables. For example, Barsky and Ahern studied the efficacy of cognitive behavior therapy for hypochondriasis (a persistent fear that one has a serious undiagnosed medical illness).[36] Clients were randomized to treatment or to usual care. The effect of treatment was measured using the Whiteley index (a measure of hypochrondriacal symptoms). Changes on the Whiteley index over time are shown in Table 11.4.

You can see that the mean Whiteley index shows that symptoms decreased in both groups over time. To test whether the decrease over time was significantly greater in the treatment group than in the control group, the investigators used repeated measures analysis of covariance; this procedure was used because the investigators wished to adjust their results for several variables, including psychiatric comorbidity, a continuous measure. The repeated measures ANCOVA showed that there was a significant interaction effect for group by time.

> Repeated measures analysis of variance and covariance require that the data meet the sphericity assumption.

Besides the other assumptions of analysis of variance (Section 3.2.C), repeated measures analysis of variance and of covariance assumes sphericity. Sphericity in a longitudinal study means that the correlation between any two measurements at different time points is the same and that within subjects there is equal variance of the measurements. (The former is similar to the assumption of an exchangeable working correlation matrix in generalized estimating equations.) The sphericity assumption is always met if you have only two measurements. But when you have three or more measurements, this assumption is often not met. Observations close in time to one another tend to be more highly correlated than observations taken far apart. Variability of the measurements tends to increase over time.

---

[36] Barsky, A. J. and Ahern, D. K. "Cognitive behavior therapy for hypochondriasis: A randomized controlled trial." *JAMA* **291** (2004): 1464–70.

TIP

Use the Mauchly test
to assess whether your
data fit the sphericity
assumption.

TIP

Use the Greenhouse–
Geisser correction
when your data do not
fulfill the sphericity
assumption.

When you have more
than one dependent
variable use
multivariate analysis of
variance or covariance.

You can use the Mauchly test to assess whether your data fit the sphericity assumption. The test is available in standard statistical software programs. The null hypothesis is that the data fit the sphericity assumption. If the P value is less than 0.05 you would reject the null hypothesis and conclude that your data do not meet the sphericity assumption. Unfortunately, the Mauchly test is very sensitive to sample size. With a large sample size, you may get a significant result even though the departure from the assumption is small, and with a small sample size you may get an insignificant result even though the departure from the assumption is large.[37]

If this assumption is not met, you can use the Greenhouse–Geisser correction. This correction reduces the degrees of freedom for the numerator; this in turn has the effect of increasing the P value. It is a conservative adjustment that makes it harder to detect differences between the groups. Therefore, if you find differences despite the adjustment you can have greater confidence that your results are robust to violations of the sphericity assumption. For example, the trial of cognitive behavioral therapy for hypochondriasis reported above used the Greenhouse–Geisser correction in reporting their results, including the results shown in Table 11.4.

When you have more than one outcome variable, you should use the multivariate forms of repeated measures analysis of variance and repeated measures analysis of covariance: multivariate repeated measures analysis of variance and multivariate repeated measures analysis of covariance. If this analysis is statistically significant, then you can look at the individual outcome variable.

One advantage of the multivariate approach is that the sphericity assumption does not need to be met. However, if you then wish to tease out the effects of the risk factors on each of the outcome variables, you will still need to test for departures from the sphericity assumption and adjust for violations of this assumption. A disadvantage of multivariate designs is that you lose one degree of freedom for each added outcome variable, making your analyses less powerful.

In general, as shown in Table 11.5., repeated measures analysis of variance is much less flexible than generalized estimating equations or mixed-effects models. For this reason, its use is declining.[38]

[37] Twisk, J. W. R. *Applied Longitudinal Data Analysis for Epidemiology: A Practical Guide.* Cambridge University Press, 2003, pp. 25–6.
[38] Gueorguieva, R. and Krystal, J. H. "Move over ANOVA: Progress in analyzing repeated-measures data and its reflection in papers published in the Archives of General Psychiatry." *Arch. Gen.*

Table 11.5 Comparison of generalized estimating equations, mixed-effects models, and repeated measures analysis of variance.

Method	Types of outcome variables accommodated	Accommodate covariates that change value during study?	Accommodate unequal number of observations?	Accommodate missing observations?	Accommodate unequally spaced observations?
Generalized estimating equations	Interval, ordinal, dichotomous, and categorical	Yes	Yes	Yes, when data are missing randomly	Yes
Mixed-effects models	Interval, ordinal, dichotomous, and categorical	Yes	Yes	Yes, when data are missing randomly	Yes
Repeated measures analysis of variance	Interval only	No	No	No	No

11.3.E Conditional logistic regression

> Clustered data with a dichotomous outcome can be analyzed using conditional logistic regression.

Clustered data with a dichotomous outcome can be analyzed using conditional logistic regression. This procedure is very similar to standard logistic regression. It produces similar outputs (e.g., coefficients, standard errors, odds ratios) and you can use similar diagnostics to assess the fit of your model.[39] In fact, "standard" logistic regression is often referred to as unconditional logistic regression. The difference between these two procedures is that conditional logistic regression takes into account the correlation between the observations.

As with standard logistic regression, conditional logistic regression does not accommodate variables that change their value during the course of the study. As implied by the name, it is a conditional technique: it produces estimates of individual-level effects conditional on membership in a cluster. Unlike mixed-effects models, another form of conditional model, conditional logistic regression cannot adjust for correlated observations owing to more than one cause (e.g., matching and clustering by sites). But when you have a dichotomous variable and observations correlated for a single reason,

Psychiatry **61** (2004): 310–7. Besides documenting the decline in the use of ANOVA methods for repeated measures, this article provides a lucid explanation of many aspects of the analysis of clustered data.

[39] Hosmer, D. W. and Lemeshow, S. *Applied Logistic Regression*. 2nd edn. New York, NY: Wiley, 2000, pp. 223–259.

conditional logistic regression may be easier to explain and perform than generalized estimating equations or mixed-effects models.

For example, Abenhaim and colleagues were interested in evaluating whether appetite-suppressing drugs cause primary pulmonary hypertension.[40] Because primary pulmonary hypertension is a rare disease with a large number of suspected but unproved risk factors, the investigators chose a matched design. Ninety-five patients with primary pulmonary hypertension were individually matched to 335 controls by age (within five years), gender, and the number of visits to the physician per year. However, beyond the variables that they used to match cases and controls, they also needed to adjust for other potential confounders including systemic hypertension, use of cocaine, and smoking status. They therefore needed to use a multivariable technique. They found, using conditional logistic regression, that after adjustment for potential confounders, use of appetite suppressants was significantly associated with an increased risk for primary pulmonary hypertension (OR = 6.3; 95% CI = 3.0 –13.2). They also showed a dose–response relationship, with subjects who used appetite suppressants for more than three months having a risk of development of hypertension 23 times greater than that of persons who did not use appetite suppressants (OR = 23.1; 95% CI = 6.9 – 77.7).

In situations where you have a choice as to which method to use to analyze data with correlated observations, you may want to analyze the data more than one way and see whether or not you get similar answers. For example, Sethi and colleagues looked at the association between the isolation of a new strain of a bacterial pathogen and an exacerbation of chronic obstructive pulmonary disease.[41] Because patients made multiple visits (81 patients made a total of 1975 visits) they needed to adjust for correlations within patient clusters. Their outcome was dichotomous: exacerbation or not. They reported similar results using conditional logistic regression and using generalized estimating equations.

> Conditional logistic regression cannot adjust for correlated observations owing to more than one cause.

11.3.F Anderson–Gill formation of the proportional hazards model

When you have censored data (Section 3.6) and an outcome that can occur more than once to a subject over time, you can use the Anderson–Gill counting process, which is an adaptation of the proportional hazards model.[42] In

---

[40] Abenhaim, C., Moride, Y., Brenot, F., *et al.* "Appetite-suppressant drugs and the risk of primary pulmonary hypertension." *N. Engl. J. Med.* **335** (1996): 609–16.

[41] Sethi, S., Evans, N., Grant, B.J.B., *et al.* "New strains of bacteria and exacerbations of chronic obstructive pulmonary disease." *N. Engl. J. Med.* **347** (2002): 465–71.

[42] Anderson, P.K. and Gill, R.D. "Cox's regression model for counting processes: a large sample study." *Ann. Stat.* **10** (1982): 1100–20.

this model subjects are considered at risk for the first event from the start of the study to the first event; they are then considered at risk for the second event from the day following the first event until the second event occurs and so on. While this gives you a method of incorporating all of the outcomes as well as all of the person-time, you still must account for the correlation between events in the same individuals. To do this use a robust variance estimate.[43]

For example, Berl and colleagues compared the incidence of congestive heart failure between patients receiving irbesartan (an angiotensin-receptor blocker) and those receiving placebo among diabetics with nephropathy.[44] Because congestive heart failure can occur more than once in the same individual the investigators used the Anderson–Gill formulation of the proportional hazards model with robust variance estimates. They found that patients receiving irbesartan had a significantly lower incidence of congestive heart failure than placebo recipients (hazard ratio = 0.72; 95% CI = 0.52–1.00; $P = 0.048$).

11.3.G Marginal approach for proportional hazards analysis

Another method for analyzing censored data with outcomes that can occur more than once to a subject over time is to model the marginal distribution of each time to outcome with a proportional hazards analysis.[45] An advantage of this approach is that the nature of the dependence of correlated observations is unspecified.

For example, Gabriel and colleagues used the marginal approach for proportional hazards analysis in a study of complications after breast implantation.[46] Most women in the study had bilateral implants; some had multiple implants in the same breast. The investigators therefore performed follow-up of each breast implant until a complication occurred, the implant was removed, or the end of follow-up occurred. Using a marginal approach to adjust for the correlation between times to implant failure for women who had more than one implant, they found that the rate of complication was significantly higher for women who had an implant for cancer or cancer prophylaxis than for those who had an implant for cosmetic reasons.

---

[43] Lin, D. Y. and Wei, L. J. "The robust inference for the Cox proportional hazards model." *J. Am. Stat. Assoc.* **84** (1989): 1074–8.

[44] Berl, R., Unsicker, L. G., Lewis, J. B. *et al.* "Cardiovascular outcomes in the irbesartan diabetic nephropathy trial of patients with type 2 diabetes and overt nephropathy." *Ann. Intern. Med.* **138** (2003): 542–9.

[45] Wei, L. J., Lin, D. Y. and Weissfeld, L. "Regression analysis of multivariate incomplete failure time data by modeling marginal distributions." *J. Am. Stat. Assoc.* **84** (1989): 1065–73.

[46] Gabriel, S. E., Woods, J. E., O'Fallon, W. M., *et al.* "Complications leading to surgery after breast implantation." *N. Engl. J. Med.* **336** (1997): 677–82.

11.4 How do I calculate the needed sample size for studies with correlated observations?

The sample-size calculations discussed in Section 6.4 assume that the observations are independent. Special methods are needed to determine sample size requirements for multivariable analysis involving clustered data.

Although these methods are beyond the scope of this text, instructions and software for calculating sample sizes for analyses of correlated outcome data are available.[47]

---

[47] Delucchi, K. L. "Sample size estimation in research with dependent measures and dichotomous outcomes." *Am. J. Public Health* **94** (2004): 372–7; Twisk, J. W. R. *Applied Longitudinal Data Analysis for Epidemiology: A Practical Guide.* Cambridge University Press, 2003, pp. 280–5.

12

Validation of models

12.1 How can I validate my models?

> A valid model is one where the inferences drawn from it are true.

> **TIP**
>
> Models rarely perform as well with new data as with the original data.

A valid model is one where the inferences drawn from it are true. Many factors can threaten the validity of a model including imprecise or inaccurate measurements, bias in study design or in sampling, and mis-specification of the model itself.

Because the development of a model maximizes the probability of obtaining the values of the original outcome data, models will not generally perform as well with new data as with the original data. This is a particularly important issue when you are creating models to predict diagnosis or prognosis and a high degree of certainty is needed.

Although predictions based on the original cases will likely not be as accurate in predicting the outcome of new cases, the important question is how large is the decrement in performance. If the decrement is small, the model is said to be validated.

The methods of model validation are:

1. Collect new data
2. Divide your existing data set:
   a. split-group
   b. jack-knife method
   c. bootstrap

Without question, the best method of validating an empirical model is to collect more data and test the performance of the initial model with the new data. This was the case with the prognostic model for estimating survival for patients with primary melanoma (described in Section 2.5). The investigators found that four factors correctly classified the vital status (alive or dead) of 74 percent of the patients. To validate their model, they studied the success of this four-variable model in predicting outcome among 142 patients who were diagnosed with primary melanoma in the same center in the two years following the enrollment of the initial sample. When applied to this new sample, the model correctly classified 69 percent of the patients, a relatively small decrement in performance from the original model.

Although testing the model with a second set of patients strengthens the validity of the model, it is not as strong a validation as testing the model on patients seen at a different center. The reason is that a model may not perform as well under a different set of circumstances (e.g., a different prevalence of disease, referral pattern, patient mix, clinician practice style, or temporal changes). In the case of the melanoma prediction rule the only difference between the circumstances of the original and the second data set was the year of diagnosis, which makes it a somewhat less rigorous validation than if the investigators had enrolled subjects from a different institution.

With a split-group validation you randomly divide your data set into two parts – a derivation set (also called a training set) and a validation set (also called a confirmatory set). The parts can be equal halves or you can split the data set such that the derivation set is larger than the confirmatory set. You develop your model on the derivation set and then test it on the confirmatory set.

A split-group validation was used to test the validity of a model designed to predict recurrence of seizures.[1] The sample consisted of 1013 people who were free of seizures on medication for at least two years. The researchers were taking advantage of an existing data set to develop a prognostic model. Collection of additional data was not an option. Instead, the investigators randomly divided their existing sample into two parts, with 60 percent of their sample in the derivation set and 40 percent in the validation sample.

Using the derivation set they developed a proportional hazards model with eight prognostic factors. To validate the model they used it to estimate the probability of a recurrent seizure for each of the subjects in the validation data set. They grouped the estimated probabilities of seizure for the patients in the validation group into eight groups of increasing probability of recurrence. As shown in Figure 12.1, for each of the eight groups they compared the proportion of actual recurrences to that predicted by the model. The bars show the confidence intervals for the predicted values, and the dash near the middle of the line shows the mean predicted value. If the validation had been perfect, all dashes would fall exactly on the diagonal line. While the dashes are close to the diagonal line, the confidence intervals are broad, especially for those predicted values where the number of subjects (shown in parentheses) is small.

> **DEFINITION**
>
> With a *split-group* validation you randomly divide your data set into two parts – a derivation set and a validation set.

---

[1] Medical Research Council Antiepileptic Drug Withdrawal Study Group. "Prognostic index for recurrence of seizures after remission of epilepsy." *Br. Med. J.* **306** (1993): 1374–8.

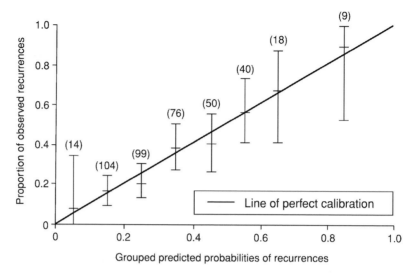

Figure 12.1   Comparison of the probability of predicted recurrences (probabilities are based on the model generated by the derivation set) to the observed probability of recurrences of seizures in the validation set. The bars show the confidence intervals for the predicted values, and the dashes near the middle of the line show the mean predicted value. Reprinted with permission from Medical Research Council Antiepileptic Drug Withdrawal Study Group. "Prognostic index for recurrence of seizures after remission of epilepsy." *Br. Med. J.* **306** (1993): 1374–8. Copyright BMJ Publishing Group.

You will note that Figure 12.1 uses essentially the same technique as Figure 8.1. Figure 8.1 is also based on comparing predicted to observed probabilities. The difference is that in Figure 8.1 the predicted and observed probabilities are based on the same subjects. In Figure 12.1 the predicted probabilities are based on a model that was derived from a different group of subjects.

One final note about validating your model using a second sample or a split sample. Once a model has been validated, investigators will often combine the multiple samples or reunite the split sample for the final model. Investigators do this so that the larger sample size can give their final model tighter confidence intervals.

In cases where it is impractical to collect more data or split your sample, you may use a jack-knife procedure (often called cross-validation). With a jack-knife procedure you sequentially delete subjects from your data set, one at a time, and recompute your model with each subject missing once. This allows you to assess two things. First, you can assess the importance of any one subject to your results. A model that substantially changes with deletion of a single case is not valid because the results hinge on that one case. Second, once

DEFINITION

With a *jack-knife* procedure you sequentially delete subjects from your data set, one at a time, and recompute your model with each subject missing once.

DEFINITION

Bootstrap procedures take random samples of the subjects in your data set with replacement and average the results obtained from the multiple samples.

you drop a case, you can predict that subject's outcome from the remaining cases. This is done sequentially such that you are predicting the values of each subject using the rest of the subjects. In this sense, the jack-knife is like a split-group validation: The split is the whole sample minus one case (the derivation set) versus the one case (the confirmatory set). When you have a relatively small sample, jack-knife procedures are likely to be more sensible than splitting your sample. You should be aware that jack-knife procedures are easy to do in multiple linear regression, but they are very computer time intensive in logistic and proportional hazards models.

The bootstrap procedure provides limited support of the validity of your model. With bootstrap procedures you take random samples of the subjects in your data set with replacement (meaning that after a case is chosen it becomes eligible to be chosen again). Thus, your random samples may include the same subject more than once, whereas some subjects will not be included at all. Once the samples are drawn, you test the strength of the relationships found in your main model in the random samples. The results from these samples can be used to construct 95 percent confidence intervals by excluding the extreme 2.5 percent and 97.5 percent of values. If the confidence intervals are relatively narrow, you can feel more confident in your results.

For example, Hamberg and colleagues used logistic regression to create a model based on clinical and laboratory data that would accurately predict cirrhosis among 303 alcohol-abusing men.[2] Such a model would have clinical significance if it decreased the need for liver biopsies. At a cut-off of 10 percent probability of having cirrhosis, the sensitivity and specificity of their model was 88 percent. They then tested their model using the same cut-off in 1000 samples drawn from their study population. The 95 percent confidence intervals for the sensitivity and specificity were 85–91 percent and 85–95 percent respectively.

Besides producing confidence intervals, bootstrap procedures produce mean coefficients and mean standard errors for your random samples. These confidence intervals and standard errors are likely to be more valid than those created from one simple model.[3]

The bootstrap procedure is a weaker test of the validity of a model than a split-group or a jack-knife. This is because the 1000 bootstrap samples of 303 subjects will have the majority of subjects in common. In contrast, a split

---

[2] Hamberg, K. J., Carstensen, B., Sorensen, T. I., *et al.* "Accuracy of clinical diagnosis of cirrhosis among alcohol-abusing men." *J. Clin. Epidemiol.* **49** (1996): 11:1295–301.

[3] Readers interested in learning more about bootstrap techniques should see: Efron, B. and Tibshirania, R. J. *An Introduction to the Bootstrap.* New York, NY: Chapman & Hall, 1993.

sample and the jack-knife procedures would have no subjects in common. Thus, in the strictest sense, bootstrap does not fit the definition of validation.

The importance of validation varies with the goals of your study. Validation is rarely performed for observational studies of etiology (Section 2.2). Your results will be judged primarily on the strength of your methods, the biologic plausibility of your results, and prior findings in this area. Other investigators may seek to replicate or refute your findings. Similarly, model validation is not generally the major issue with interventional trials, in which, it is naturally assumed that the results need to be replicated in different populations, even if no multivariable modeling is performed. In contrast, models predicting diagnosis or prognosis of disease (Sections 2.4 and 2.5, respectively) are rarely published (at least not in the best journals) without validation.

The reason for the distinction is that models used to determine factors associated with a particular outcome do not need to be highly accurate. For example, while exercise is significantly associated with mortality, the decrease in mortality owing to exercise is relatively small. You certainly would not try to predict a patient's life span based on knowing how much he or she exercises. But that's not the point. The point is that, in a population, exercising will result in increased longevity for the group as a whole. Improving risk factor profiles may have a substantial effect on the development of disease in a large population, even if the absolute effect for an individual is small. This is especially true if the disease and the risk factor are common.

In contrast, with studies designed to predict diagnosis or prognosis, a high degree of certainty is required because you are using the model to predict for an individual patient. Clinicians are not likely to trust a model that has not been validated. (Even then, physicians are notorious for ignoring diagnostic algorithms, preferring instead their gut instinct; see Section 2.4.)

TIP

Clinicians don't trust models that are not validated.

Special topics

13.1 What if the independent variable changes value during the course of the study?

DEFINITION

Time-dependent covariates allow incorporation of changes in the independent variables that occur during the study.

Let's say that over the course of a longitudinal study a subject's value changes on an independent variable. This may happen because the patient quits (or starts) a habit such as smoking, begins a new medicine, or develops a new symptom or illness. How can you deal with this in your analysis? The answer is that within proportional hazards analysis you can create time-dependent variables. These variables change value at a particular point in time. So, instead of having a variable such as smoking at baseline (yes/no), you create a time-dependent variable, where each subject is 0 (nonsmoker) or 1 (smoker) at a particular point of survival time.

In the simplest case, time-dependent variables change their value only once (e.g., a nonsmoker starts to smoke – the variable is 0, 0, 0, at several points in time before the subject begins smoking and then the variable changes value to 1 at the time the subject begins smoking and remains 1 for the remainder of the observational time). It is also possible to construct time-dependent variables that change their value back and forth multiple times (reflecting what sometimes happens when smokers try to quit). Time-dependent variables need not be dichotomous; that is, the variable may take the value of an interval measure, such as blood pressure, at each point that it is measured.

While the interpretation of time-dependent variables can be complicated, their construction is easy. You need to look up the exact formatting in your statistical package, but in general, the package will have a special designation for time-dependent variables. You tell the computer when (in study time) each subject changes value on the variable.

13.2 What are the advantages and disadvantages of time-dependent covariates?

The advantage of time-dependent covariates is that you can incorporate important events that occur during the course of the study. For example,

Mayne and colleagues wanted to determine if depression shortened survival of HIV-infected men.[1] Their subjects were part of a longitudinal study that began in 1984 with more than seven years of follow-up. The simplest design for answering this question would be to measure depression in 1984 and then follow subjects longitudinally for mortality. The problem with this design is that depression may not be present initially (in 1984) but may develop subsequently. Using depression at baseline only will weaken your study (because people who become depressed six months after baseline will not be considered depressed in the analysis, even though this may affect their mortality). Second, using depression only at baseline decreases your power because relatively few persons will be classified as depressed at one time. Third, a single instance of a participant being rated as depressed might not affect mortality, since it might reflect only a short episode of depression, rather than a more chronic condition.

To overcome these issues, the researchers created a time-dependent variable that took the value of the proportion of visits at which the person was depressed. So for each visit (subjects were interviewed every six months) the variable had a value between 0 percent and 100 percent (of visits to date) at which the person was depressed. They found that depression was associated with a higher rate of mortality. They also created time-dependent variables that represented each subject's actual score on the depression index at each visit. The results were similar.

The depression measure was not the only variable that changed value over the course of this study. The subjects' immune function also changed value as patients progressed. The investigators therefore created time-dependent covariates that represented the subjects' CD4 counts, as well as other measures of immune function. They found that depression increased the risk of death, even with adjustment for changes in immune function. This would suggest that the mechanism of depression on mortality is not mediated by more rapid immune function decline (within the limits of the investigators' ability to measure it). This analysis also weakens an "effect–cause" hypothesis (that participants became depressed because they learned of their CD4 count results), since the analysis adjusts for recent CD4 counts.

Another advantage of time-dependent covariates is that they do not have to fit the proportionality assumption (Section 3.6). The reason is that they incorporate time and therefore do not have to be independent of time.

---

[1] Mayne, T. J., Vittinghoff, E., Chesney, M. A., *et al.* "Depressive effect and survival among gay and bisexual men infected with HIV." *Arch. Intern. Med.* **156** (1996): 2233–8.

The disadvantages of time-dependent covariates are less obvious than the advantages. The two major disadvantages are: overadjustment and decreased usefulness of the model for clinicians.

Adjusting for prognostic markers that are on the pathway to your outcome may prevent you from identifying the effect you are investigating (overadjustment). Let's go back to the example of depression and mortality in HIV-infected persons. Assume that the overall finding is accurate, that is, that depression increases mortality. But, let's assume that the mechanism by which this happens is that depression leads to worsening immune function, which, in turn, leads to more opportunistic infections and death (in other words, change in immune function is an intervening variable between depression and mortality) (Section 6.3). If this is the case, then including time-dependent variables measuring immune function will eliminate the effect you are trying to substantiate. Depression will not be associated with mortality because adjusting for changes in immune function will eliminate the effect. In comparison, if you adjust only for immune function at baseline you will not eliminate the effect.

The use of time-dependent covariates may also decrease the value of your models for clinicians. The reason is that clinicians must advise their patients based on information they have at the time they are counseling the patient. A clinician can't know how a risk factor will change in the future. It would be confusing to a patient to counsel them on their risk of heart attack in case they *were* to develop hypertension at a particular time in the future.

With time-dependent models it is important to include only events that have occurred before the outcome. Remember that an advantage of a longitudinal design compared to a cross-sectional one is that a longitudinal study is more likely to support causality. That's because if the outcome is not yet present (at least, as best as can be measured), the chance that the "outcome" causes the "risk factor" (i.e., effect–cause) is much less likely. (Remember, in a cross-sectional study you are measuring risk factors and outcomes at the same time.) With time-dependent variables, you are including factors that are more proximal to outcome than baseline measurements. Thus, effect–cause becomes a greater danger. One way to deal with this issue is to "lag" the time-dependent measure substantially before the outcome (but still after the baseline).

A lag for time-dependent variables was used by the investigators to see if depression would still be associated with mortality if the depression measure was lagged by periods of one, two, and three years from the outcome. With these time lags, depression was still associated with mortality, supporting the hypothesis that depression increases mortality, and weakening

TIP

With time-dependent covariates include only events that have occurred before the outcome.

the case for the alternative hypothesis that depression reflects worsening health status.

13.3 What are classification and regression trees (CART) and should I use them?

Classification and regression trees (CART), also known as recursive partitioning, is a technique for separating (partitioning) your subjects into distinct subgroups based on the outcome.[2]

The technique is easiest to follow visually. In Figure 13.1, you see an algorithm for assessing the risk of heart attack that was developed using CART.[3] The algorithm is based on 1379 patients, of whom 259 (19 percent) had a heart attack. The investigators assessed the diagnostic ability of 50 variables, including patients' history, physical examination, and electrocardiogram results.

The CART technique attempts to divide the sample into subgroups that have as many patients with the outcome (e.g., heart attack) in one group (high risk) and as few patients with the outcome in the other group (low risk). You can see that at the first branch point of Figure 13.1 (ST elevation or Q waves in two or more leads, not known to be old), CART separates the sample into two groups with very different probabilities of heart attack: 80% and 9%. At the next branch point (chest pain began ≥48 hours ago), the sample is also separated into two groups with different probabilities of outcome (10% vs. 3%), although this difference is not as large as the difference in the first branch point. Selecting from the candidate variables, CART will continue partitioning until it reaches a point where it is no longer possible to partition the sample into subgroups with distinctly different risks of outcome. If your CART model partitions your sample into subgroups where the risks are not sufficiently distinct, you can prune your tree back.

What advantage does CART have over other multivariable techniques? It is similar to forward stepwise logistic regression in that you are estimating a dichotomous outcome by sequentially choosing the strongest risk factors for your outcome. The major difference between CART and forward multiple logistic regression is that with CART one branch can have different risk factors for outcome than a different branch. With multiple logistic regression your risk factors are for your entire sample, not one branch of it. For this reason,

[2] See the bible of CART: Breiman, L., Friedman, J. H., Olshen, R. A., *et al. Classification and Regression Trees*. Pacific Grove, CA: Wadsworth & Brooks, 1984, p. 189.
[3] Goldman, L., Cook, E. F., Brand, D. A., *et al.* "A computer protocol to predict myocardial infarction in emergency department patients with chest pain." *N. Engl. J. Med.* **318** (1988): 797–803.

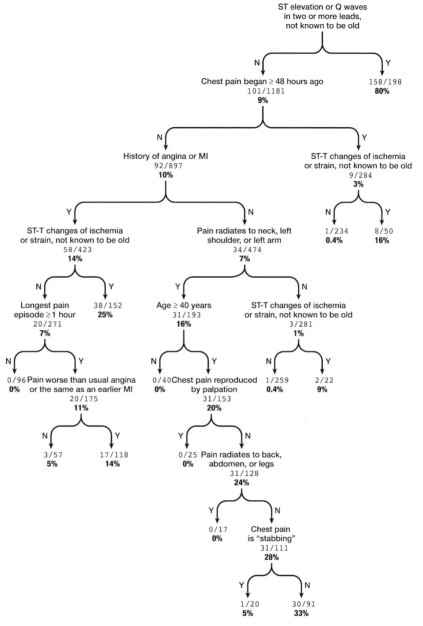

Figure 13.1   Classification and regression tree for predicting the likelihood that the patient has a myocardial infarction. The data are from Goldman, L., *et al.* "A computer, protocol to predict myocardial infarction in emergency department patients with chest pain." *N. Engl. J. Med.* **318** (1988): 797–803. The figure is adapted from Lee, T.H., *et al.* "Ruling out acute myocardial infarction." *N. Engl. J. Med.* **324** (1991): 1239–46. Copyright (c) 1991 Massachusetts Medical Society. All rights reserved.

The major difference
between CART and
forward logistic
regression is that with
CART one branch can
have different risk
factors for outcome
than a different
branch.

CART is better suited to data where there are interactions (because with inter-actions a variable may be important for only a portion of the sample) (see Sections 1.4, 7.3, 8.4, and 9.7).

An advantage of diagnostic trees is that compared with multiple logistic regression they more closely reflect how physicians make decisions. Certain pieces of information take you down a particular diagnostic path; you seek more information to prove or disprove that you are on the right path. Most clinicians do not, in their mind, total up all the information, positive and negative, and make a decision.

Having said that, clinicians have shown no greater willingness to adopt this decision rule than that of Pozen and colleagues (Section 2.4). When the authors attached their prediction tree to the back of the patient data forms in their own hospital, physicians looked at it in only 46 percent of the cases; in the 115 cases in which the prediction rule was used, it changed the triage decision only once. Moreover, the likelihood of using the rule decreased with increased level of physician training (i.e., interns used it more than residents, who used it more than attendings). This is despite the fact that the decision model shown in Figure 13.1 was shown to perform better than physicians at university and community hospitals when tested prospectively.

One disadvantage of the chest pain model is the large number of variables it includes. A widely used algorithm that was developed using CART predicts whether or not a patient has an ankle fracture based on only three variables.[4] The model, referred to as the Ottawa ankle rules, has a sensitivity of 100 percent for predicting fracture. Therefore, patients who are negative on the decision rule do not need to be sent for an x-ray film. This saves a great deal of money and time for the patient. The lower specificity of the model (50 percent) is not a major problem because at one time practically all patients with an ankle injury would have received an x-ray.

Because of their convenience and high sensitivity, the Ottawa ankle rules have received much wider acceptance than the heart attack prediction models. This should not, however, be taken as a negative reflection on heart attack prediction models. It is not surprising that it takes more variables to accurately predict a heart attack than a broken ankle, and that even with a large number of variables, there is greater uncertainty in the prediction of a heart attack than a broken ankle. It does highlight, however, that

---

[4] Stiell, I.G., Greenberg, G.H., McKnight, D., *et al.* "Decision rules for the use of radiography in acute ankle injuries: Refinement and prospective validation." *JAMA* **269** (1993): 1127–32; Stiell, I.G., McKnight, R.D., Greenberg, G.H., *et al.* "Implementation of the Ottawa ankle rules." *JAMA* **271** (1994): 827–32.

clinicians are more likely to adopt diagnostic rules that are simple and have high sensitivity.

13.4 How can I get best use of my biostatistician?

Working with a biostatistician should be an iterative process, a dynamic interaction between the clinical details and the statistical realities of your study.

With a complicated study, a biostatistician should be consulted at each phase of the analysis. At the design phase, review with a biostatistician the statistical implications of different study designs and seek their help in conducting or reviewing your power calculation. After conducting your univariate and bivariate data analysis, discuss with your biostatistician strategies for dealing with skewed distributions, nonlinear relationships, multicollinearity, and missing data. Based on the preliminary analysis, determine together the best type of multivariable analysis to perform. Finally, once you have your multivariable model, review it with your biostatistician so as to assess whether the model fits. At this stage a review of the residuals may be particularly helpful.

You will find that all biostatisticians are not alike. Some are primarily interested in developing new methods of analyzing data (data at the service of methods). Others are interested in using methods for improving the analysis of the data (methods at the service of data). In general, you will do better if you have the latter type of biostatistician, although we wouldn't have so many useful statistical techniques if it were not for the former type.

Just as it helps to know more about your car in dealing with car mechanics, the more you know about your research project, and the statistical issues surrounding it, the more helpful your biostatistician will be to you. Or, to switch to a medical metaphor, think of yourself as the primary care doctor and the biostatistician as the specialist.

13.5 How do I choose which software package to use?

Almost all of the popular statistical packages (SAS, SPSS, BMDP, STATA, S-PLUS) perform the same types of analyses. The best one to choose will probably depend on what others in your research group use. Programming questions invariably arise and it is always helpful to have other users nearby.

As with foreign languages, some statistical packages are harder to learn than others, but once you know one it is easier to learn others. While I have not performed any formal polling, most medical researchers use SAS. On the one hand, SAS is somewhat more difficult to learn than the others, in part, because the manuals are poorly organized and confusing. On the other hand, SAS is more flexible and powerful than most of the others. The flexibility is particularly important for longitudinal studies, where you have multiple observations of the same person. The SAS package also allows you to write your own statistical programs, but it also costs more than some of the others. The STATA package is running a close second to SAS in popularity because it can perform many of the same analyses of complicated longitudinal data as SAS (e.g., generalized estimating equations) but is easier to learn and use.

Some packages are particularly good at certain functions. The S-PLUS package has dramatically increased in popularity because it has fantastic graphing capabilities. R (http://www.r-project.org) is modeled after S-PLUS and is free, making it an excellent choice if you are doing research on your own with a tight budget. The software package MlwiN was specially created to perform multilevel models (Chapter 11). It is available free (http://multilevel.ioe.ac. uk/download/index.html) on the Internet. The SUDAAN package is often chosen for analyzing weighted data sets.

14

Publishing your study

14.1 How much information about how I constructed my multivariable models should I include in the Methods section?

The editors of the major biomedical journals have developed guidelines on how much detail of the statistical analysis to include in manuscripts. While the guidelines are general, the editors articulate an important rule of thumb: "Describe statistical methods with enough detail to enable a knowledgeable reader with access to the original data to verify the reported results."[1]

Although that goal is important, anyone who has performed statistical analysis knows that it would be impossible to include every detail of the analysis in a manuscript. Imagine writing: "for each independent variable we assessed whether there was any difference in outcome between the 'don't know' category and the 'missing' category" or "for one variable, we found that there was a somewhat increased frequency of outcome in the 'don't know' versus the 'missing' category, so we …" I think you get the idea. Research requires thousands of decisions. The readers rely on you to make the right ones. It is your responsibility, however, to report on the important choices you made, especially those that influence the results.

Published articles and journals differ in how they organize the information in the Methods section. I prefer dividing the Methods section into a review of how subjects were enrolled (Subjects), what interventions were used or how data were acquired (Procedures), how the variables were coded (Measures), and how the data were analyzed (Statistical analysis). But some published

---

[1] International Committee of Medical Journal Editors. "Uniform requirements for manuscripts submitted to biomedical journals." *Ann. Intern. Med.* **126** (1997): 36–47 (also available at www.icmje. org); See also: Moher, D., Schulz, K. F., Altman, D., *et al.* "The CONSORT statement: Revised recommendations for improving the quality of reports of parallel-group randomized trials." *JAMA* **285** (2001): 1987–91; Des Jarlais, D. C., Lyles, C., Crepaz, N., *et al.* "Improving the reporting quality of nonrandomized evaluations of behavioral and public health interventions: The TREND statement." *Am. J. Public Health.* **94** (2004): 361–6. For an excellent guide on writing up your research for publication see: Browner, W. S. *Publishing and Presenting Clinical Research.* Philadelphia, PA: Lippincott Williams and Wilkins, 1999.

articles group all of the information under a general heading of Methods. Before writing this section for your manuscript, consult a recent issue of the journal to which you plan to submit your paper; you will get a sense of the journal's preferences. At a minimum, include a description of the following in your Methods section:

1. The population from which your subjects were chosen and your method of choosing them (e.g., probability sample of households in low-income census tracts, consecutive sample of patients presenting to a specialty clinic with sinusitis).
2. Your sample size. If any sampled subjects were excluded, explain why (e.g., three subjects were excluded because of insufficient blood samples).
3. Response rate, including differences between persons who participated in your study and those who did not. (Some journals prefer that this information be reported in the Results section.)
4. Nature of intervention (e.g., patients were randomized to one of three arms of drug therapy), if applicable.
5. How data were acquired (e.g., interviews, matches with registries).
6. How your independent and dependent variables were chosen and measured.
7. How your independent and dependent variables are categorized in the analysis (e.g., nominal, multiple dichotomous variables).
8. What bivariate statistics you used (e.g., chi-square statistics for categorical variables, t tests for interval variables).
9. What type of multivariable model you used (e.g., multiple linear regression, conditional logistic regression).
10. How you dealt with missing data.
11. What independent variables were eligible for inclusion in the model (e.g., all variables listed, those independent variables associated with the outcome at $P < 0.15$).
12. If you used a variable selection procedure, state type (e.g., forward, backward) and what the inclusion/exclusion criteria were (e.g., $P < 0.10$).
13. If you had censored observations, when you censored them (e.g., alternative outcomes, date of the end of the observation period).
14. How you tested the linearity assumption for interval-independent variables.
15. How you tested the proportional odds assumption for proportional odds regression.
16. How you tested the proportionality assumption for proportional hazards model.

17. Whether you tested for interactions and, if so, how.
18. What statistical software you used. (The reason for this is that some packages differ in their computational methods for certain statistics.)
19. Whether *P* values were one- or two-tailed.

Within the Methods section, my preference is to report 1–3 in the Subjects subsection, 4 and 5 in the Procedures subsection, 6 and 7 in the Measures subsection, and 8–19 in the Statistical analysis subsection; but, journals and reviewers vary in their preferences.

14.2 Do I need to cite a statistical reference for my choice of method of multivariable analysis?

There are two reasons for providing a citation for the type of analysis you are performing:

1) To provide a source for interested readers who are unfamiliar with the procedure you are performing and want to learn more
2) To defend your method of analysis in an area where there is controversy concerning the best way to perform your analysis

There are no hard-and-fast rules about which procedures need explanation beyond the name of the procedure, in part because the sophistication of readers differs by journals. However, it is certainly unnecessary to cite a reference for multiple linear regression and logistic regression. Some people provide a citation for proportional hazards regression and it is usually the same classic citation:

Cox, D.R. "Regression models and life tables." *J.R. Stat. Soc.* **34** (1972): 187–220.

However, I don't see the value of this type of citation because this classic article would not be the right place for a beginning reader to go to learn about this procedure – it is too complicated, and explanations of proportional hazards analysis are easy to find in statistics textbooks. On the other hand, if you were writing an article using Poisson regression and/or negative binomial regression for an audience that is unfamiliar with these procedures it may be helpful to cite a general article that addresses these techniques specifically:

Gardner, W., Mulvey, E.P., and Shaw, E. "Regression analyses of counts and rates: Poisson, overdispersed Poisson, and negative binomial models," *Psych. Bull.* **118** (1995): 392–404.

When you are performing an analysis that is both unfamiliar and may be controversial, it is often helpful to provide a reference. A reference can both support your choice and help readers to obtain more detail about how you set up your analysis without your including a long description in the statistics section, which is often difficult given the word limits of most journals. For example, it may be helpful to provide a reference for the method used for assessing the proportionality assumption of proportional hazards regression or for why you chose a particular working correlation matrix for generalized estimating equations.

14.3 Which parts of my multivariable analysis should I report in the Results section?

As with the question of what to include in the Methods section, there are no absolute rules on what results to report in your published paper.

Unless there are no missing data, you should report the n for each analysis. For multiple linear regression models, most investigators report the regression coefficients, the standard errors of the coefficients, and the statistical significance levels of the coefficients. As a test of how well the model accounts for the outcome, most researchers report the adjusted R^2.

For logistic regression and proportional hazards analysis, even though the coefficients are similar to those from linear regression, they are not generally reported. Instead, report the odds ratio or relative hazard and the 95 percent confidence interval. The latter incorporates information from the standard error and the P value, and so it is not necessary to report these as well. Reporting on how well the model fits the data is variable. Some authors will report the likelihood ratio test or the Hosmer–Lemeshow test, or they may compare the estimated to observed probabilities of outcome in graphical or tabular form, or they may do none of the above (Section 8.2.B). For diagnostic or prognostic studies, some measure of prediction (sensitivity, correctly identified cases, c index) will usually be provided (Section 8.2.B).

There is an increasing tendency for clinical researchers to show only the results from the main variables of interest. This is illustrated in Table 14.1, reproduced from a study of the risk of cardiovascular disease and stroke in women.[2] The investigators assessed, using proportional hazards analysis, whether current estrogen or current estrogen/progestin increased the risk of coronary artery disease or stroke.

---

[2] Grodstein, F., Stempfer, M. J., Manson, J. E., *et al.* "Postmenopausal estrogen and progestin use and the risk of cardiovascular disease." *N. Engl. J. Med.* **335** (1996): 453–61.

Table 14.1 Relative risk of cardiovascular disease among current users of conjugated estrogen alone or with progestin as compared with nonusers, 1978 to 1992.

Hormone use	Person-years	No. of cases	Major coronary disease Relative risk (95% CI)		No. of cases	Stroke (all types) Relative risk (95% CI)	
			Age adjusted	*Multivariate adjusted* [†]		*Age adjusted*	*Multivariate adjusted*[†]
Never used	304 744	431	1.0 (ref.)	1.0 (ref.)	270	1.0 (ref.)	1.0 (ref.)
Currently used							
Estrogen alone	82 626	47	0.45 (0.34–0.60)	0.60 (0.43–0.83)	74	1.13 (0.88–1.46)	1.27 (0.95–1.69)
Estrogen with progestin	27 161	8	0.22 (0.12–0.41)	0.39 (0.19–0.78)	17	0.74 (0.45–1.20)	1.09 (0.66–1.80)

[†] The analysis was adjusted for age (in five-year categories), time (in two-year categories), age at menopause (in two-year categories), body-mass index (in quintiles), diabetes (yes or no), high blood pressure (yes or no), high cholesterol level (yes or no), cigarette smoking (never, formerly, or currently [1 to 14, 15 to 24, or 25 or more cigarettes per day]), past oral-contraceptive use (yes or no), parental history of myocardial infarction before the age of 60 years (yes or no), and type of menopause (natural or surgical).

Reprinted with permission from Grodstein, F., *et al.* "Postmenopausal estrogen and progestin use and the risk of cardiovascular disease." *N. Engl. J. Med.* **335** (1996): 453–61. Copyright © 1996 Massachusetts Medical Society. All rights reserved.

In the published table, the investigators report the person-years, the number of cases of outcome for the analysis, the relative risk (I would prefer the term relative hazard), and the 95 percent confidence intervals. The relative risk was adjusted first for just age and then for numerous other variables that affect the likelihood of coronary disease and stroke. These variables are listed at the bottom of the table next to the cross sign. Although each of these variables has a relative risk and a 95 percent confidence interval, these values are not presented. Based on other studies, we know that some of the variables listed at the bottom of the table (e.g., age, smoking) are significantly associated with coronary artery disease and stroke.

The advantage of not showing the relative risks and confidence intervals for these variables is that these results would take up a whole page. Also, this study was designed to show the influence of estrogen and estrogen/progestin use on coronary artery disease and stroke. It was not designed to estimate the effect of age or cigarette smoking on these outcomes. Other studies have answered these questions.

However, there are disadvantages to showing your data in this way. The reader cannot assess whether the impact of estrogen and estrogen/progestin use on coronary disease and stroke is as strong (or stronger) as other factors, such as smoking. Second, your study may be less helpful to future researchers. For example, if someone was doing a meta-analysis on the effect of past oral-contraceptive use (a variable that has been inconsistently related to outcomes such as coronary disease and stroke) they wouldn't learn anything from the table. You don't know whether oral contraceptives are or are not related to the outcomes in this study.

Finally, when evaluating a published report, one feels greater confidence if the independent variables operate in ways you would expect them to based on prior research. For example, if the investigators reported that cigarette smoking was related to coronary artery disease and stroke it would give you confidence that their model was sound. Conversely, if smoking was not related to these outcomes you would worry about the validity of their model.

All this being said, demands and cost of journal space are likely to dictate more presentations of data like Table 14.1. With large models, and multiple independent variables, it is hard to show all the results. One solution to this dilemma is gaining in popularity: Investigators inform readers where they can obtain the full analysis (usually by contacting the authors or by accessing the journal's website). This seems a good balance between publishing extensive tables and having results available to the public.

TIP

If you are unable to publish your full analysis, make a detailed version of your results available on the web.

15

Summary: Steps for constructing a multivariable model

Step 1. Based on the type of outcome variable you have, use Table 3.1 to determine the type of multivariable model to perform (if you have repeated observations of your outcome see Table 11.2).

Step 2. Perform univariate statistics to understand the distribution of your independent and outcome variables. Assess for implausible values, significant departures from normal distribution of interval variables, gaps in values, and outliers (Section 3.2C).

Step 3. Perform bivariate analysis of your independent variables against your outcome variable.

Step 4. If you have any nominal independent variables transform them into multiple dichotomous ("dummied") variables (Section 4.2).

Step 5. Assess whether interval-independent variables have a linear relationship with the outcome (Section 4.3). If not, transform the variable, use splines, or create multiple dichotomous variables.

Step 6. Run a correlation matrix. If any pair of independent variables are correlated at > 0.90 (multicollinearity), decide which one to keep and which one to exclude. If any pair of variables are correlated at 0.80 to 0.90 consider dropping one (Chapter 5).

Step 7. Assess how much missing data you will have in your multivariable analysis. Choose a strategy for dealing with missing cases from Table 6.4.

Step 8. Perform the analysis (Chapter 7).

Step 9. Assess how well your model fits the data. (e.g., F test, likelihood ratio test, adjusted R^2, Hosmer–Lemeshow test, c index) (Section 8.2).

Step 10. Assess the strength of your individual covariates in estimating outcome (Section 8.3).

Step 11. Use regression diagnostics to assess the underlying assumptions of your model and to determine strategies for improving the fit of the model (Chapter 9). For proportional odds regression make sure the proportional odds assumption is met (Section 9.8); for proportional hazards models, be sure that the proportionality assumption is met (Section 9.9).

Step 12. Decide whether to include interaction terms in your model (Sections 1.4, 7.3, 8.4, and 9.7).

Step 13. Consider whether it would be possible to validate your model (Chapter 12).

Step 14. Publish your results in the *New England Journal of Medicine* and be the envy of your friends and colleagues.

If you have questions or suggestions for future editions send them to me at mhkatz59@yahoo.com.

Index

additive assumption, 171–3

Aerobics Center Longitudinal Study, 2, 5, 7, 54

alpha, 98, 107

analysis of covariance (ANCOVA), 30–2

    repeated measures, 200–3

analysis of variance (ANOVA), 26–32, 35–6

    assumptions, 32–5

    one-way, 29

    repeated measures, 200–3

ANCOVA. *See* analysis of covariance

Anderson–Gill counting process. *See* counting process

ANOVA. *See* analysis of variance (ANOVA)

antilogarithmic transformation, 80

arcsine transformation, 35

assumptions, 162–79

    additive, 171–3

    censoring, 50–8

    equal variance, 32–5, 68, 165–6, 202

    linearity, 76

    logistic regression, 78

    multiple linear regression, 32–5, 165–6

    multiplicative, 171

    normality, 35, 68, 165–6

    proportionality, 58–60, 174, 176–9

    proportional odds, 42, 174

    sphericity, 202–3

backward selection, 136–8

bell-shaped distribution, 32–4

best subset regression, 137

beta, 98, 149. *See also* coefficient

bias, 10, 15, 17–19, 52, 109–10, 131–2, 194

binomial distribution, 38, 114

biostatistician, 74, 97–8, 162, 219

bivariate analysis, 3–4, 8–9, 15–17, 25–7, 33–4, 40, 44–5, 93–5, 97–8, 108–10, 134–5

BMDP, 219

Bonferroni correction, 159–60

bootstrapping, 208, 211–12

c index, 146–7

CART. *See* classification and regression trees (CART)

case-control study, 9–10

categorical variable, 29–32, 36, 74, 98–9. *See also* nominal variable. *See also* dichotomous variable

causality, 1–2, 14, 187

censoring, 46–51, 54, 127–8

    and alternative outcome, 51–2

    and loss to follow-up, 50–1

    and study withdrawal, 52–4

    and varying time of enrollment, 54–5

    assumptions of, 50–8

    end point, 55

    nonrandom, 56

    validity of, 55–8

central limit theorem, 35

change score, 191–2

chi-squared, 40, 42–3, 79, 153–5, 169

    distribution, 142–3

    homogeneity, 11

    model chi-squared. *See* likelihood ratio test

    trend, 36

classification and regression trees (CART), 216–19

clustered observations, 194, 198, 207

    and matching, 204–5

    and multiple body parts, 185, 198

coefficient, 12, 149–61

    correlation, 26–8, 40, 89–90, 191

    multiple linear regression, 149–51

    of variation. *See* R^2